M

TOXIC WORK

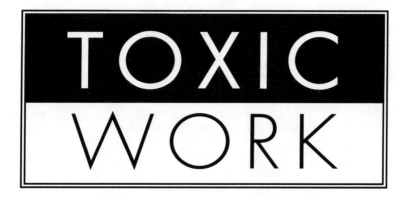

TOXIC WORK

HOW TO OVERCOME STRESS, OVERLOAD, AND BURNOUT AND REVITALIZE YOUR CAREER

Barbara Bailey Reinhold, Ed.D.

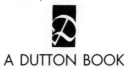

A DUTTON BOOK

DUTTON
Published by the Penguin Group
Penguin Books USA Inc., 375 Hudson Street,
New York, New York 10014, U.S.A.
Penguin Books Ltd, 27 Wrights Lane, London W8 5TZ, England
Penguin Books Australia Ltd, Ringwood, Victoria, Australia
Penguin Books Canada Ltd, 10 Alcorn Avenue,
Toronto, Ontario, Canada M4V 3B2
Penguin Books (N.Z.) Ltd, 182–190 Wairau Road,
Auckland 10, New Zealand

Penguin Books Ltd, Registered Offices:
Harmondsworth, Middlesex, England

First published by Dutton, an imprint of Dutton Signet,
a division of Penguin Books USA Inc.
Distributed in Canada by McClelland & Stewart Inc.

First Printing, May, 1996
10 9 8 7 6 5 4 3 2 1

 REGISTERED TRADEMARK—MARCA REGISTRADA

LIBRARY OF CONGRESS CATALOGING-IN-PUBLICATION DATA:
Reinhold, Barbara Bailey.
Toxic work : how to overcome stress, overload, and burnout and revitalize your career /
Barbara Bailey Reinhold.
p. cm.
Includes bibliographical references and index.
ISBN 0-525-93875-3
1. Job stress. 2. Employee empowerment. 3. Vocational guidance.
4. Work—Psychological aspects. 5. Work—Physiological aspects.
I. Title.
HF5548.85.R444 1996
650.1—dc20   95-26490
CIP

Printed in the United States of America
Set in Times New Roman and Futura
Designed by Eve Kirch

This book is printed on acid-free paper. ∞

For Sandy Lovejoy

CONTENTS

ACKNOWLEDGMENTS

I have many people to thank for different kinds of support through this long, two-year process of simultaneously working full-time and writing a book. To my extended family, who many times felt that we should set a separate place at the table for the writing project that had moved in, I am apologetic, and I am grateful for their patience and support. I'm also grateful to the entire staff of the Smith College Career Development Office, who gracefully endured the pulls of my double life and were constantly on the lookout for resources for me.

People too numerous to list were idea-generators, readers, cheerleaders, and editors for the seemingly endless versions of the manuscript along the way to publication: among them were Jana Zvibleman, Renee Hill, Jane Sommer, Laurie Shannon, Carrie Hemenway, Alan Goldberg, Suzie Rheault, Joan Laird, Ann Hartman, Cheryl Pinkham, Ferna Shrewsbury, Virginia Vernon, Suzanne Slater, Julia Demmin, Felice Schwartz, Penny Locey, Geoffrey and Greta Reinhold, Bonnie Bailey Baker, Dr. Charles Brummer, Dr. Lucy Hann, Dr. Philip Livingstone, Dr. Les Jaffe, Dr. Josef Arnould, Linda Workman, Margie Kolchin, Gaynelle Weiss, Kathleen Chatwood, and the Nag's Heart group. Two colleagues were present every step of the way—Robin Kinder and Joanne Murray, both of whom gave most generously of their expertise and expended hours neither one could really spare from her own busy professional life.

My partner Sandy Lovejoy was ever-present, helping to launch and fine-tune the idea, editing and contributing important concepts, and doing the hard work of managing the preparation of the manuscript. She is truly the co-architect of this project.

I'm grateful to Carole DeSanti, editorial director at Dutton, who introduced me to the world of publishing and who was a generous, patient, and witty mentor, particularly in the final breathless stages of the project. John Paine was also very helpful in the dense middle part of the editing. It was an honor to have two such excellent wordsmiths on my side.

INTRODUCTION

An estimated twenty million Americans are staying in jobs they hate in order to keep their health insurance—when research indicates that career dissatisfaction is more likely than anything else to make them need to use it. Polls have shown, moreover, that less than 10 percent of Americans are really satisfied with their work. Are you satisfied? Do you feel that your work is not merely a job but an enhancement to your life, to your health and well-being? You deserve to.

In your own workplace, you have probably heard (and perhaps even made) some of these despairing comments:

- "The work just keeps on piling up—and makes me want to scream."
- "It's depressing to be in that shut-down environment."
- "I hate not having time for a life."
- "This job doesn't use my talents."
- "I've been stuck here for twelve years, and there's just no place for me to go."
- "My boss treats us all like children."
- "My job doesn't mean much to me anymore."
- "It's time for me to be on my own now."

For twenty-five years I've been counseling and teaching people of all ages about the negative effects of being in work that has become "toxic." Engineers, lawyers, doctors, mechanics, secretaries, writers, shopkeepers, judges, and other counselors have come to me for help in figuring out why they felt depressed, anxious, devalued, or angry about their work situations. People suffer for a variety of reasons. Some problems, such as unreasonable managers and business upheavals, are organizational. Others are due to discrepancies between individual workers' needs and their employers' requirements. Some people found that their dream jobs looked good, but *felt* terrible. Others were in jobs they once enjoyed but had since outgrown.

During the late 1980s, in addition to my counseling practice, I was often called into corporate and nonprofit work units as a consultant/trouble-shooter, to find out why people were having difficulty working together productively and managing work teams. What I saw in these work places impressed me deeply and made me listen to my clients in a whole new way. I realized that people frequently punctuated their descriptions of work concerns with references to *physical* complaints and health problems. I began to hear comments like these:

- "This fall schedule is a backbreaker."
- "That new project is a killer."
- "My manager is such a pain."
- "There's just no room to breathe around here."

Stories like these often sounded like segments from a health-care call-in show. It became clear to me that not only did jobs distress people emotionally, but they also caused physical problems. Ever since, when people have pained expressions on their faces while describing their work, I ask, "Where in your body does this pain reside?" And people usually know: "Right in the gut," "It's the stiffness across my shoulders," or "This headache just won't quit," they say. Once the connection between physical pain and job stress has been made, symptoms can be seen as signals for change, and a different kind of dialogue begins. It is that dialogue that became a central theme of my work and the subject of this book.

Some attention has been paid elsewhere to literally toxic jobs, those involving chemical fumes, radiation, and so on. But another kind of "toxic work" has been almost totally ignored. This is the gap between what people needed to stay engaged and healthy at work and what most jobs actually involved.

Work May Be Hazardous to Your Health

To understand why workplace difficulties were causing so many physical as well as emotional symptoms, I began a journey of reading, researching, and interviewing a variety of mainstream and alternative health-care practitioners. As I explored, a world of physical, emotional, and spiritual interdependence opened. There was no escaping the fact that work has profound effects on emotions and health.

As a nation, we have focused great concern on our health-care system, yet we often ignore one of our greatest health risks: the way we do our work. For example, we've known for more than twenty years that the greatest predictor of heart attacks in people under fifty—more potent even than smoking, high blood pressure, elevated cholesterol, or diabetes—is job dissatisfaction.[1]

Sometimes, just *thinking* about going to work can be lethal. Statistically, more people have heart attacks and strokes on Mondays, between eight and nine a.m. than at any other time of the week. The relationship between work stress and cardiovascular emergencies is so clear that it's been given a special name: Black Monday Syndrome.[2] We know that many other bodily symptoms are affected by work, too. At Boeing Aircraft, for example, researchers found that lower back pain was much more likely to occur in workers with low job satisfaction, whether they were in physically demanding blue-collar jobs or working at a desk.

In fact, career stress is the single greatest health problem for working adults, according to Paul Rosch, president of the American

Institute of Stress. And the economic, as well as human, costs are staggering. In 1994, stress cost more than $300 billion. In California, the cost of stress-related illness increased more than 800 percent in a decade. But despite all this evidence, most organizations have yet to address the problem in any comprehensive or organized way.

And recent changes in the nature of American work have raised the stress level of many workers to new heights. Many current stresses arose because we did not prepare adequately for the complexities of dual-career families or for the cost-containment moves and the loss of low-skilled jobs that globalization and automation have brought. As one "outplacement" consultant remarked to me, "Not since the Industrial Revolution have our assumptions about work been so turned on their heads."

It's no wonder that workers frequently tell me they're scared; fear is a realistic reaction to the economic roller-coaster ride of the 1990s. Millions of jobs have been lost in the past decade, and people are well aware that the bloodletting isn't over yet. A 1994 *New York Times* poll found that three of four people interviewed had lost a job or benefits in the recent past, or were close to someone who had. And for every person who actually lost a position or benefits, many more spent months agonizing about whether the ax would fall on them.

What's more, work environments will never be stable in the old predictable way again. Fewer than 15 percent of families have the luxury of having one wage earner and one support person at home to keep the ship afloat. On average, Americans aged thirty-five to forty are only half as wealthy as their parents were at a comparable age. Low-skill manufacturing jobs are moving offshore to places like Pakistan and Thailand, where workers can be hired for $500 per year. The epidemic of "reinventing government" and defunding nonprofit organizations has created whole new categories of unemployed people. We are also moving inexorably toward an unsettling new ratio of permanent to temporary employees. By the end of the century, it's estimated that less than half the labor force will work full time for one employer. The rest will be part-time, seasonal, or contract workers, responsible for designing and choreographing their own careers and retirements.

Although some organizations are making changes to improve workers' quality of life, there's still much to be done in the American workplace.

You Can Detoxify Your Life

So where does this leave you, who might have grown up with one set of career expectations and are now knee-deep in another set? Where does it leave you if you are hanging on in a "stable" job situation that doesn't address certain important needs in your life? And what are you to do about those stress-induced headaches and back pains?

While you cannot control some events (such as organizational decisions to sell, merge, or downsize), you can control how you *react* to those events. You can also control the *impact* of your own feelings of discontent on the rest of your life. Two major things make the difference: how you *interpret* what's happening at work, and whether you are able to see life's upheavals and dissatisfactions as *catalysts* rather than *catastrophes*.

As a career-counseling professional, I know that work doesn't have to make you sick. For decades my clients and I have sorted through the myriad problems that toxic workplaces present, and we've found some interesting solutions. I'll share them with you in the chapters that follow.

Before I could help others, though, I had to clear up some job confusion of my own. During one period of change in my ever-evolving career, I paid a visit to Jungian analyst Alice Howell for a career consultation of my own. I was having trouble fitting the range of things I enjoyed into a single job description, and the kind of career counseling I was drawn to do didn't conform to the field's conventions. After hearing me out, she put a name to the work I wanted. "You're a *permissionary*," she said. "Your life's work is giving people *permission* to find and do the things they really want to do, no matter what other people expect of them." And with this new (though strange-sounding) notion, I proceeded to help my clients replace the "I should's" in their lives with "I can's" and "I want to's." My philosophy has always been "If the 'should' doesn't fit, don't wear it." Somehow we find more "shoulds" in the area of work than in almost any other part of life.

I've found that giving clients permission to follow a dream or leave a toxic situation has powerful effects. People have found ways to escape ill-fitting jobs, start training programs, or enter graduate school. Others created enterprises of their own or designed patchwork careers, weaving the threads of their skills and passions into a tapestry of several part-time jobs. Still others realized that they wanted to do the same kind of work, but needed to change how they did it.

Staying in a toxic job is especially sad because work is one of the greatest potential health *enhancers* we have. Doing a good job and being appreciated for it builds self-esteem and sense of purpose, which in turn enhances functioning of the cardiovascular and immune systems. Many studies show that work satisfaction increases both health and longevity. Positive work situations are also more likely to provide good relationships and new learning, both of which medical research has shown to be correlated with staying healthy.

So you, like most American workers, are probably at a major crossroads in your life. You can learn sound strategies for staying healthier and more productive within this permanently uncertain work environment, or you can suffer a great deal of emotional and physical pain. In *Toxic Work*, I will help you explore ways to create positive change from difficult and challenging situations.

Toxic Work will help you pinpoint the workplace predicaments and stressors that are particularly harmful to you. It will also suggest actions you can take on your own and with co-workers to make your work a health enhancer rather than a sickening factor in your life. I've seen incredible triumphs over seemingly impossible situations and potential career disasters. Lives *can* change, and careers *can* be revitalized. The choice is yours.

PART I

RECOGNIZING
AND MANAGING
TOXIC WORK

1. The Toxic Workplace

Most of the solutions advanced to address stress . . . address only its symptoms. Little is done to change the source of the problem: work itself. While we recognize that stress is damaging, we act as though its sources were inevitable.

—ROBERT KARASEK

Harvard Business School professor Louis "By" Barnes believes in having honest dialogue about life in organizations. When he spoke to a group of senior administrators during a major organizational reconfiguration at Smith College several years ago, many were shocked to hear him say, "From the perspective of individual employees, the organization will almost always betray them at some point."[1]

Betrayals, Broken Covenants, Bad Management

Much has happened over the past few years to confirm the veracity of Barnes's admonition, in all kinds of organizations. "Betrayal" by organizations has become a common occurrence. If you work at management level, perhaps you've noticed that the language in memos and meetings has changed. In the 1980s, the talk was all about developing, nurturing, and growing. Once the downsizing fever began to spread, however, consultants analyzing language changes in organizations discovered that words like "take out," "kill," and "terminate" outnumbered the expansive vocabulary words six to one. Through all of this, some workers have pretended that things could stay the same. One author described employee denial in downsizing organizations this way: "They believed 'til the door hit them in the ass on the way out."[2] For many employees, the changes have been experienced as the kind of blow Barnes was describing.

So how deep is this sense of betrayal? At General Electric, one of the premier American corporations, two out of every three layers of management have been eliminated, and the workforce reduced by almost half. In early 1994, nationwide and across all industries, more than 3,100 workers were dismissed each day. Eighty-five percent of Fortune 1,000 companies handed out pink slips between 1987 and 1994, while Fortune 500 firms sloughed off a quarter of their workers.[3] Organizations are currently laying off 2 million workers a year. In their wake, "survivors" struggle with gargantuan workloads and shrinking rewards. For many people, *that* spells betrayal. We have also lost more than 20 percent of manufacturing jobs, traditionally the safest route to good wages for non–college graduates. Despite the fact that only one-third of downsizing companies have realized increased profits from this hemorrhaging of jobs, the cuts are expected to continue. What's more, as productivity and profits have soared in the past five years, real hourly wages have fallen. Labor's share of the largesse is lower than it has been for three decades. The upshot of all this is that more than three-quarters of corporations interviewed in a study by the American Management Association reported deteriorated employee morale.

Whether we want it to be true or not, the traditional employer-employee covenant has been shattered by permanent changes in the shape and speed of work. Products once languished for years in development; it took fifteen years to move television from the drawing board into our living rooms. Now many new-product developers have barely the luxury of fifteen weeks to get a product designed and off to market. You need to be able to move swiftly, changing gears and learning new skills without complaining. You also need to be able to do other people's jobs as well as your own. Indeed, many of the jobs we had are gone, while new ones are evolving all the time. But the responsibility for ferreting out new opportunities in the hidden job market and for having the cutting-edge skills to make the most of them is yours.

Another complication of the nineties is that many organizations that were willing to be flexible and trusting in easier economic times have somehow fallen into an anxiety-ridden mode of self-protection. It is seldom the official policy of an organization to be mistrusting, deceitful, or exploitative in its approach to its employees. Nonetheless, that seems to be happening in many places. And when that happens, the atmosphere becomes toxic for everyone, including those in charge. Against the backdrop of an enormous allocation of resources for executive development and management training, this epidemic of bad management is particularly hard to fathom.

That's what brought Ellen, a hardworking and ambitious woman in her mid-thirties, to see me. Ellen worked in human resources in a mid-sized manufacturing facility, where she was the employee-development specialist. According to her job description, her role was to conduct ongoing assessments of staff training needs, working primarily with supervisors in different work teams. During the hiring process, she had also been assured that she'd be able to meet directly with employees periodically, to be sure that the company's training program reflected the perceived needs of both managers and workers. And so she had begun the job more than a year earlier feeling optimistic about launching an energetic educational program for the organization, a goal she felt was strongly endorsed by senior management.

When Ellen arrived for her counseling appointment, she kept her upper-respiratory inhaler in hand as she told me about the differences between what she had expected in her job and what was actually happening. In her view, an essential covenant had been broken. She described major cutbacks in her training budget and a series of meetings in which her boss had decided against surveying employees about what training they felt they needed. She then went on to describe her boss's need to know everything that went on in the company. He monitored mail and computer communications, attendance records and phone logs to find out where people might be deviating even slightly from company policy.

On the boss's shelf sat the usual management journals, full of articles about teamwork and participatory management and the central role of training and retraining in keeping organizations competitive—all to no avail, as far as Ellen could tell. Many managers, like Ellen's boss, who find it hard to trust in people or open-ended processes are finding it hard to navigate the choppy seas of this turbulent economy: trying out new strategies of inclusion and participation for employees in uncertain times can feel like learning to sail in a hurricane. And so Ellen, like many other workers, was suffering from the discrepancy between senior management's vision of the larger organization and her own supervisor's terrified, dictatorial hand on the tiller.

Eventually, I asked Ellen how long her asthma had been bothering her. About six months, she said, ever since she had realized that her boss had no intention of letting her do the job she thought she had been hired to do. Ellen's physical symptoms hadn't developed overnight. There had been other signals along the way. But she was ever the "good employee," and tried to pretend that nothing was wrong. Finally, reality intervened. Ellen persisted in trying to perform as directed, but her body decided to make the messages impossible to ignore.

Ellen is not alone. Walter is a prematurely graying man in his early forties, dressed impeccably in a well-tailored suit. He holds himself stiffly because of the constant pain in his upper back. "There's always this terrible pressure and weight on my shoulders," he explains as he talks about his job as executive director for a major human-services organization. "An impossible boss is one thing, but twelve impossible bosses, like the members of my board, who can't get along with each other, who don't know what to do about the impending funding cuts, and who then take it out on me, is just too much. The rules change with every meeting, and then I have to go back and tell staff members that the ultimatums we got last meeting have changed to new ones. Everybody groans and we start over. No wonder we have so much absenteeism in the office." Like so many others in organizations where disapproval, diminution, and negativity permeate the atmosphere, Walter has also felt his own health and vitality gradually slip away from him over the past several years.

Karen is also in pain. She works as controller in a large architectural firm in which the CFO has just decided to outsource the management information systems function. Karen has watched what happened as the MIS director was let go and external managers came in and changed the rules for people who had worked there for years. Morale in the MIS unit is hovering around zero, but nobody at the top seems to be noticing. In fact, the rumor is out now that the CFO is considering outsourcing purchasing and accounting as well, and she wonders what this means for her. The CFO plays her cards rather close to her chest, however, and so Karen feels she can only wait and wonder. That's the fearful, passive stance she's taken for the past four months, working many extra hours to "show how important I am to the organization," and suffering one bout of bronchitis after another.

Bernard's mantra these days is "I didn't quite have time." Since his promotion from high school principal to superintendent of the local school system eight months ago, Bernard has put on nearly forty pounds. "I just seem to eat my way through one stress-filled day after another, starting with community breakfasts and ending with late school committee dinners," he says woefully. He has begun to wonder if he's just not good enough for the job, because he puts in more than eighty hours most weeks, and still can't stay on top of things. Of course, it has been an incredible year so far—school funding was cut by nearly 12 percent, causing him to lay off teachers and eliminate successful programs that he had worked hard to build when he had been a principal.

"I didn't create all these programs just to tear them down," he said to his senior staff when the word about the funding cuts first came down, but he has had to do just that. He has also broken up with the woman he hoped to marry—"You're already married to your job," she told him as she left—and his other friends have similarly grown tired of waiting for his call. The Bernard I see here today is lonely, exhausted, and having trouble keeping it all together.

Then there's Rob, a creative, industrious software engineer who has been hired and fired twice now in one year, for reasons totally unrelated to his performance. A year ago he was recruited from his large, somewhat stodgy organization to help develop a new line of products for a start-up company. His enthusiasm for his colleagues and the new products allowed him to blink at the company's first profit-and-loss statements as they rolled in. Four months into the venture, his great new bosses gave the entire division the boot—"Sorry, the time's just not right for those products now." But Rob was smart, well-connected, and a little bit desperate to keep his gargantuan mortgage going, so it took him only five weeks to snag a job with another firm, this time a large one like the one he had left. But now he's just heard that the trial-balloon line the company had floated has been edged out in the market by a similar product with more bells and whistles, and so guess what? Everybody's sorry all over again. And how is Rob feeling? He's pretty mad and still desperate about his mortgage. He's also finding it hard to walk around or sit for long because of lower back pain.

Let's look at someone younger. Emily has been out of college for five years. At first she thought the boredom was about having to "start at the bottom" and work her way up in the publishing firm that had recruited her right after graduation. "The bottom is the pit," she murmured to herself more than once during her first year or so. She was smart and competitive, and so in time the promotions came as planned. With each new title her hours got longer, but the tasks didn't get any more challenging. It was all the same old stuff, with very little real meaning and no intellectual "ah-*hah*s" like the ones she remembered from college. But she didn't dare complain about her work or her constant tiredness, because her standard of living had stealthily escalated to the point where with each raise and bonus she barely kept ahead of her debt. "I'm an indentured servant to my credit cards," she moaned to friends at her college reunion last spring. Now she's been diagnosed with Chronic Fatigue Syndrome and can't get out of bed some days.

Some of these testimonies have to do with stressors that employers are inflicting on people. Others are about personal, individual reactions to one or more aspects of work. In most cases, it's an interactive event: something problematic is happening at work that goes against the person's own style or agenda. Certainly the exhaustion of Bernard, the superintendent of schools, has as much to do with his own personal style (his inability to manage his time well, his compelling need to be liked and appreciated, and his perception of himself as a builder of programs rather than a maintainer of the bottom line) as with the difficult hand he's drawn in the game of school funding. But attitudes and behaviors that might have been a tolerable nuisance in less turbulent times have become career- and health-threatening now. Bernard and the others, as well as most of you, would do well to spend some time sorting out the "inside" and "outside" factors making people susceptible to the ravages of toxic workplaces.

What Makes Work Toxic?

Disease or dysfunction is the body's way of saying that we have failed to adapt, adjust, or change to meet the situation or that we have done so at the price of physical or mental disturbance. —BLAIR JUSTICE

The syndrome of toxic work overtakes you when what's happening to you at work causes protracted bouts of distress, culminating in emotional suffering or physical symptoms and heightened by the perceived inability to stop the pain and move on to find or create a more rewarding situation. Feeling stuck where you are, unable to imagine or take your next steps, is perhaps the most debilitating part of the problem.

For some people, it was apparent from the start that a job didn't fit. But because of financial desperation or pressure from family members or others, they've stayed on, becoming more and more worn down. For others, the awareness of displeasure sets in gradually. It can creep up in the aftermath of changes in the job or in the environment of the office or plant. Still others simply outgrow the work they've done for years. Whatever the cause, toxic work situations sap your energy and lull you into a stupor. Then the insidious eating away of energy and self-esteem begins in earnest. This is the end result of toxic work: it makes you collapse in on yourself, just when you need most to be involved in structured, purposeful activity to prepare to make a change.

Of course, some of us react to workplace stress by denying there's a problem, and exhausting ourselves in the process. Denying is shutting down in some way, trying to tell yourself (and your body, which is not about to be fooled) that this assault is not happening. The end result is a little like leaving your headlights on all night and expecting the car to start in the morning. Even people who should know better have ended up paying a price for denying what they are feeling. For instance, researchers in a twenty-five-year study headed by Caroline Bedell Thomas asked thousands of bright, high-achieving graduates of the Johns Hopkins School of Medicine how they dealt with problems, as they were leaving medical school and periodically during their medical practice. The research revealed that those who kept things bottled up inside themselves developed fatal cancer of all types at greater rates than their more attentive and expressive colleagues.[4]

The denial process has in fact become part of workplace toxicity. We use a variety of anesthetics to keep ourselves from knowing what we're thinking and feeling. You may be someone who reaches compulsively for whatever keeps your mind off troubling situations at home or work: painkillers, tobacco, food, recreational or prescription drugs, gambling, shopping—and work. Working harder to keep yourself from knowing there's something wrong for you at work is baffling, ironic, and incredibly common!

Many people suspect their work may be making them sick, and yet they ignore it. Rather than greeting physical symptoms as signals from their unconscious minds or intuitive messages about their own needs, they bludgeon their symptoms into submission with one form of anesthetic or another—a response somewhat like going around the house ripping out all the smoke detectors. It's testimony to how we react to pain that we've welcomed more than four hundred new analgesics onto pharmacy shelves in the past several years. But denial will not do: if your work is making you sick, it is imperative that you put the anesthetics back on the shelf and attend to some *real* work, right now.

It's Up to You: Choices in the Toxic Workplace

There is the risk you cannot afford to take, and there is the risk you cannot afford *not* to take. —PETER DRUCKER

Against the backdrop of economic crisis and organizational responses, Professor Barnes's admonition about betrayal rings true. It's hard not to experience these changes either as personal affronts or as extraordinary demands made without adequate preparations or appreciation. So what do you do? Should you work harder in the same old ways and hope for the best? Give up and be depressed? Or just tune out altogether?

None of those solutions work, not for very long at least, because Barnes's words about betrayal actually have more to do with you than with your employer. Perceived betrayals of various sorts can be devastating. That's understandable. But here's the rub: when you choose to hang onto feeling betrayed, you give away your own badly needed power. Toxic work situations present you with important choice points, which in turn have a major impact not only on your career, but, more broadly, on the degree of emotional and spiritual maturity you attain. Neither maturity nor wisdom can be purchased except through making hard choices and learning from highly challenging experiences. No matter how difficult it seems, you can learn to use the offending situations as catalysts for taking control of your own life. Consider the following three *choice points* lurking in most toxic work situations:

- Balance or overload?
- Autonomy or self-doubt?
- Engagement or alienation?

Balance Versus Overload: Are You Having a No-Life Crisis?

Personal issues must take a central role as business objectives; they cannot be relegated to the margins without negative repercussions for both employees and their employers. —LOTTE BAILYN

Starting in the early eighties, the Japanese began to notice a syndrome called *karoshi*: sudden death by overwork. Highly successful salarymen (the Japanese name for professionals and managers) began dropping dead at their desks, usually just after the completion of a particularly tense or demanding project. More than ten thousand workers each year have succumbed to this syndrome of excess. Once they had deduced the relationship between work overload and this epidemic of sudden deaths, the Japanese government set up a *karoshi* hot line, which receives thousands of calls. In an even bolder move, officials designated November 22 as "National Couples Day," hoping to encourage Japanese workers to bring their lives into better balance.

But still, thanks in part to the cool reception that corporations gave these reforms, Japanese employees persist in working eleven-hour days on average and in taking less than half of their allotted vacation days. And this is the model so often held up to Americans as the ideal by shortsighted organizations seemingly unaware of the unhealthy outcomes and the diminished productivity that the Japanese themselves are now trying to modify. It's interesting to note that a 1991 study by the Organization for Economics Cooperation and Development revealed that American workers are 60 percent more productive than their Japanese counterparts. This is so, analysts suggest, in large measure because so many American companies are coming to understand that business objectives and employee satisfaction are inextricably linked.[5]

Still, in many organizations, American workers are affected by impatient, often relationship-deprived Type A personalities, who seem unaware of the need for employees to have balanced lives. They breed half the emergencies themselves by their "do it yesterday" mentality. Then they overreact to the ones they didn't cause, spewing out the contagion of anxiety and stress all around them. People who are more comfortable with working than they are with other aspects of life end up buying into the workaholic norms in organizations, contributing to what Juliet Schor has called our epidemic of "time poverty."[6] A deadly resoluteness often overcomes people who take their work so seriously that they leave no time for play or rest.

I remember a conversation with a man who informed me that his life was much better since he had "discovered" a new way to balance his professional and personal life. Ed worked until six p.m. and then went home to have supper with his wife and kids. So far so good. Ed helped put the kids to bed between eight and nine, then napped himself for several hours. At midnight, he got up and went back to the office and worked all night, returning home again at six a.m. After a shower, breakfast, and seeing the kids off to school, he went to work again. "It's a great improvement," he told me. "Most weeks I only have to do it two or three nights to stay caught up." This was by some standards a clever solution, I suppose, were it not for the fact that exhausted people are seldom able to perform at consistently high levels or with sufficient creativity to meet new challenges. Nor are they able to keep their relationships (and hence themselves) healthy. Relationships require time to keep on growing—even though the average working couple currently spends only twenty minutes a day sharing time together.[7]

The research of Boston psychologist Rosalind Barnett is critical here. In her studies of three hundred dual-earner couples, she found that both men and women in good relationships were able to withstand workplace stress better than people who tried to deal with difficult work situations without that support.[8] Another surprising study, by Peter Capelli and his colleagues at the Center for Human Resources at the Wharton School, found that those males and females graduating from high school in 1972 who said that they valued having a strong family life earned more money over the next fourteen years than their classmates who didn't.[9] Both of these studies call into question the prevailing notion that work and relationships must always be pulling at opposite ends of the rope.

My own research with Smith College alumnae is applicable here. In the aftermath of the media fascination with Felice Schwartz's article on women's careers in the *Harvard Business Review*, my colleagues and I surveyed nearly seventeen hundred women in a range of fields and at different levels in organizations. Eighty-nine percent of the mothers in the sample reported that their parenting experiences had made them more effective at work. In particular, they believed that they had developed critical managerial strategies such as coaching, staying calm in crisis situations, and rewarding incremental improvements in performance. When men and women can transform their view of relationships from "role conflict" to "role enhancement," workers, families, and organizations will all benefit.

Stephen Covey, in his book *The 7 Habits of Highly Effective People*, advises that you must keep your *productive activities* and your *production capability* in balance. When you work at full tilt constantly, without time for relationships, rest, and regeneration, you compromise your ability to stay maximally effective in your job. Neither you nor your boss can afford to forget that you are like a high-quality machine—you need to be treated well in order to keep on producing at maximum capacity.[10] Few people would purchase an expensive automobile and then neglect to service it, but some don't give a second thought to the kinds of service a person needs in order to stay healthy and do his or her job well. Certainly the midnight-to-dawn executive wasn't paying much attention to how to keep his *production capability* strong.

If your supervisors are not tuned in to the ameliorative effects of parenting and other good relationships on work performance, however, you may be in the position of having to educate the people to whom you report. I've seen groups of workers take on that project with success. They have employed such strategies as proposing articles for the company newsletter, bringing in speakers for seminars, or petitioning their human resources departments to run training programs for managers. They also have formed support groups intent on ensuring that managers in their departments see whatever articles or programs they can find about the interrelationship of balanced lives and worker effectiveness. Changing someone's attitude is slow work, however. Most of my clients don't have time to wait for their bosses to see the light: they need to make some decisions now, while their kids are young and their relationships are still intact.

In my years of working with employees and their supervisors, I've observed what happens to managers who have allowed their own lives to get out of balance. The supervisors who are the least flexible and understanding of the need for balance in their employees' lives are usually the ones who need more balance themselves. Somehow, however, their response to that unspoken need has been to get angry and vindictive when the people who report to them ask for time off to be with family members, to have some relaxation, or even to recover fully from an illness. So if you're a supervisor who finds yourself getting bent out of shape frequently at the lack of commitment to the job your direct reports seem to be showing, it's very likely a sign that you need to be choreographing some new dances in your own life.

Autonomy Versus Self-Doubt: Do You Really Have Control?

The most stressful workplaces are those where a demanding pace is coupled with virtually no individual discretion.
—JULIET SCHOR

Work also becomes toxic when you feel that things are out of control, for one reason or another. For a century now, American industry has been dutifully applying the techniques of Frederick Taylor, the "father of scientific management." Taylor's time studies did indeed bring both a sense of order and an appreciation for the need to train and value workers. He got manufacturers to streamline processes and develop standard expectations for manual labor. His emphasis on predictability was helpful and appropriate then, when there was little order in factories and mills and when the workforce ran more on brawn than brainpower. Management guru Peter Drucker, in fact, sees Taylor as having had as much influence on history as Karl Marx or Sigmund Freud.[11] But Taylor's insistence on the kind of control that comes with narrowly defined jobs is disastrous in our volatile information and service economy. Research shows clearly that the control we need now can only come from inviting workers to be more autonomous, helping to shape and reshape their own jobs in response to rapid market changes.

Quantum theorist Erich Jantsch advises us that "in life, the issue is not control, but dynamic connectedness."[12] Management theorists have moved in exactly that direction. But for a generation of managers who came of age practicing structured Taylor techniques for spelling out quite specifically how workers should do their jobs, letting go of the "how to get there" part of charting a course is tough, even severely counterintuitive for many of them. Unfortunately, organizations need to do just that in order to harness the creative power of their employees. The most successful organizations have figured out how to offer their employees a clear sense of direction and then empower them to design their own work.

Even the National Institute for Occupational Safety and Health has recognized that overly regulated management styles affect workers' health. Incidents of "Stuffy Building Syndrome" at NBC and New York University in New York City are telling evidence of the physical potency of feeling out of control at work. In both situations, employees were moved into new, hermetically sealed work spaces, whereupon they began to report a range of physical symptoms, such as dizziness, sore throats, headaches, fatigue, and burning eyes. When health inspectors investigated, they found no problem of physical toxicity. But they did identify problems with how jobs had been designed and how people were being managed. When workers were given a chance to "air" their grievances and implement strategies for how their jobs got done, the physical symptoms disappeared.[13]

According to researcher Robert Karasek, the worst thing that can happen to workers, in terms of both productivity and health, is to have high demands—which almost all workers do these days—but low control over how they meet those demands. When employees are in positions where they have little opportunity to use their own judgment in fulfilling the requirements of their jobs or varying the pace of their activities, they are at risk for various physical and emotional maladies. Karasek's work on what he calls "low decision latitude" shows that both heart disease and reduced creativity result. He suggests that "if instead jobs could be redesigned with high decision latitude—that is, with opportunities for taking responsibility through participative decision-making—demands would be seen as challenges, and would be associated with increased learning and motivation, with more effective performance, and with less risk of illness."[14]

His research blamed high-demand/low-control jobs for a range of cardiovascular illnesses in both American and Swedish workers. But that's not the only combination. When you have low control coupled with low demands, your work will not be particularly impressive. Neither will your health, because you'll be bored and not very involved. But when the demands are high and your control over how the work is done is high also (and if your work still seems to "fit," which we'll discuss later), both your productivity and your health benefit. This in turn feeds your sense of accomplishment and your self-esteem, and increases the likelihood of success and good health in the future. To what degree is that positive cycle of challenge and autonomy happening for you in your work now?

Another way to help employees feel self-direction rather than self-doubt is to let them know what's really going on and what they might expect to happen, particularly when things seem to be changing so radically in many organizations. Consider what a difference appropriate sharing of information can make. In a study by psychologists Ellen Langer and Susan Saegert, two groups of women were sent to high-traffic supermarkets at peak shopping time with long shopping lists. One group was given no information except to fill their baskets with the items on the list and get to the checkout counter as quickly as possible. The second group, however, was warned about the possible effects of crowding in the aisles during the exercise, and told that if they got anxious they should simply stop, breathe deeply a few times, and then keep going. Nervousness and some confusion were "normal" during experiments like these, they were assured, and nothing to worry about. At the end of the exercise, there were distinct differences in the performance of the two groups. The "informed" group got more shopping items correct, were more satisfied with the store, and felt less stressed than the "uninformed" shoppers.[15] Perhaps some of your physical and emotional symptoms might be alleviated by more information about what's really going on at work, and what you might be able to do about it.

Yet another aspect of worker control is the idea of "employability": taking responsibility for the shape and motion of your own career. Employability is the notion that employers no longer can promise job security—but they will instead offer you opportunities and resources for you to develop new skills in order to keep yourself employable.[16] Within the framework of employability, rather than waiting for your manager to alter your job description, deploy you to some new task, or suggest that you upgrade particular skills, it's your job to be talking to him or her about what tasks and projects you'd most like to be doing—now and in the future. Some economists have gone so far as to suggest that organizations ought to put workers squarely in charge of their own careers, giving them ITAs (individualized training accounts), rather than IRAs, to force them to design their own long-term career training and retraining.

Like some current tax proposals, ITAs would provide tax incentives for workers to seek out retraining and education, in anticipation of continued restructuring in organizations. Potentially, this could decrease the number of workers requiring unemployment compensation and make a huge difference in the self-esteem and sense of autonomy of employees in volatile organizations. My own theory has long been that the only real job security is your perceived ability to walk away to something else. But nobody will provide that for you. You have to get it for yourself, by updating your skills constantly and staying alert to new opportunities. Smart employers will help you do that, because they know that their most capable workers, the ones they really need in these competitive times, are the ones who know how to look out for themselves and keep on growing.

Research clearly shows that feeling out of control, in one way or another, is dangerous to your health. Clients have shown me that, whatever the cause, the absence of self-directedness inevitably feeds a creeping self-doubt. As employees feel themselves hemmed in, they become frustrated and angry. If they stay too long in situations that they perceive to be denying them respect and limiting their opportunities to influence the shape of their own workdays, they lose confidence in themselves. This feeling in turn hardens into lack of interest in work. The end result, then, is a lose-lose situation for both the organization and the employee. The organization has a less productive worker and the employee gets to wrestle with a series of physical and emotional problems.

Engagement Versus Alienation: Fight, Flight, or What?

When you feel connected to something, that connection gives you a purpose for living.   —Jon Kabat-Zinn

Fight or flight—aren't those the choices? Some people stay and fight after enduring an organizational betrayal of one form or another. They write stinging letters, they confront people at meetings, they patrol the place sniffing out more injustices, and they sometimes threaten legal action. This may feel good at first, but because reputation is such a critical component of organizational life, once you get known as too independent or "testy," maintaining status or real power in that organization is virtually impossible. What's more, we know that unrelieved anger will soon take its toll on your cardiovascular health.

The alternative seems to be flight. Quite understandably, most workers who are feeling betrayed instinctively withdraw at first. Sometimes they choose to lick their wounds in quiet or stay in a shut-down state, raging inwardly for years. Some people put a permanent protective distance between themselves and the betrayal. One problem with withdrawal, however, is that it leads to a state of psychological and physiological disengagement in which you experience a slowing of vital reactions. As a team of University of Rochester researchers discovered, "When we overdo the reaction and become virtually unresponsive to everything around us, physiological changes may occur that place us at risk for illness or even death. It is as if we have carried playing possum too far, held our breath too long, or hibernated to such an extreme that there is no return."[17]

So what is the choice? If neither fight nor flight will work in the long run, how are workers who feel betrayed supposed to survive, emotionally and physically? Research from wartime is useful here: it's healthier to be active rather than passive in difficult times. During World War I, for example, American troops who were actively engaged in battle stayed healthier than those in less danger back in base camps. During the Korean War, members of attacking companies, who felt a greater sense of activity and purpose than those in defending companies, also took only half as long to shake off the physical effects of stress.[18] When you feel betrayed by an organization you once trusted, it can feel like a kind of war—with "friendly fire" from your own side. But the same maxims apply. Reengaging in one way or another is the approach most likely to keep you well.

A look at the data unearthed in an eight-year study of executives at Illinois Bell after the AT&T divestiture also shows how important it is to stay connected. In fact, some people even manage to thrive in potentially stressful situations. Researchers Salvatore Maddi and Suzanne Kobasa Ouellette coined the term *psychological hardiness* to describe the qualities that they found differentiated those executives likely to get sick from those who stayed well during this organizational upheaval. Three qualities characterized those employees who stayed the most healthy (in fact, seven times as healthy) during that period of uncertainty:

- *Challenge:* They saw the enormous task of reconfiguring Illinois Bell as a personal and organizational opportunity rather than as a disaster.
- *Control:* They believed they had the power to make things come out all right in the end, for themselves and for the organization.
- *Commitment:* They maintained strong bonds and emotional ties to their organizations or to the field, as well as to their families and communities.

The managers who reported the most illness, on the other hand, felt panicked, powerless, and alienated, even though they were in exactly the same situations as the "hardy" executives.[19] The message from Maddi and Ouellette is that it's not the stress itself, but rather what you do with it, how you interpret it to yourself, that makes all the difference.

There are lots of ways to give away your power without even knowing you're doing it. Another way is by sliding into a "victim" stance. Maddi and Ouellette found, for instance, that some of the executives had wives who were too willing to commiserate and who encouraged their husbands to feel mistreated and stay mad at the company, and that those executives failed to recommit to the organization and do the mental shifts necessary to get themselves moving again. The problem was not having angry feelings—it was staying stuck there. As a result, the executives with the doting wives exhibited both lower productivity and more health problems than their colleagues who were able to express their feelings and then move forward. So advise your supporters that you may need their help to get yourself reconnected to the organization in some way and moving through the problem—not so much for your employer as for yourself.

Is There Any Hope?

If a human being is not allowed to grow with his cultural environment, then he must of necessity grow against it.
                                    —George Lockland

So what happened to the six toxic-work sufferers we met at the
beginning of this chapter? All of them found ways to reduce the
toxicity and to regain their health and improve their productivity.
Let's look at their cases in more detail.

First, Ellen, the corporate training specialist: The first step in
helping Ellen make some decisions about her toxic workplace was
to ask her to sit back, put her hands in her lap, get comfortable, and
take several slow deep breaths. Gradually, her hunched-over shoulders straightened and the tension lines around her mouth and eyes
softened. After guiding her into a relaxed state with her eyes closed,
I asked, "What would you need at work each day to be able to
breathe more easily? Say each thing out loud as it comes to you and
I'll keep a list." It was important to have her close her eyes, so she
could locate and rummage around in her less obedient, more natural
urges.

After she finished, I asked her to open her eyes so that we could
talk about what she had identified. As we talked, I read aloud from
the list of fourteen items she had named, everything from "someone
to have relaxed lunches with" to "a chance to ask employees about
what management skills their supervisors need most."

Then we considered each item on the list. Ellen made a best
guess as to how likely each one was to happen in the current situation. Reluctantly, at the end of the exercise, Ellen saw that only
four of the items were even remotely possible. She sat stunned. After that, it didn't take her very long to decide that she really did
need to leave the company as quickly as possible. She would need
to do some networking. Fortunately, a regional conference of the
American Society for Training and Development was scheduled for
the next month. Because she hadn't been feeling well, Ellen had decided not to go. That decision was reversed on the spot. Of course
she had to go, not only to learn what was happening in other orga-

nizations, but also to renew old contacts and make some new ones to help her in her search.

In six months of some intensive networking, Ellen was able to find another training position, this time in a large nonprofit organization that was glad to get someone with varied corporate experiences. "It means about a fifteen percent pay cut," she noted when we last met, "but I can breathe again. When you factor in the savings in extra doctor visits and prescriptions, I think I'm breaking even."

What about Walter, the aching executive director who was being harassed by his inexperienced board of directors? The first thing Walter did was get his life in order. He told the board and his staff that he needed to take two weeks of his seldom-used vacation time in order to rest, collect his thoughts, and come back with a plan to get things under control. Once he had a few days at his family's mountain lake retreat to pull himself together, Walter realized that it wasn't worth destroying his health and family life to stay with a job that was bringing him mostly grief. So he decided to make one last try at improving communication. If that didn't work, he promised himself, he would be on his way.

He arrived back at work tanned and rested, feeling better than he had in years, and announced calmly but forcefully to the board that he would resign immediately unless they agreed to make some changes. The changes included working with outside consultants to restructure the organization so that it could respond better to the funding crises weighing it down. The board, it turned out, was relieved to be offered the option of some outside expert advice, and agreed to a year's contract for the consultants to work with them devising and implementing the organization's first strategic plan. Now that Walter had the strength and presence of mind to be leading differently, the board somehow responded differently too.

Several important things happened. The consultants recommended a reprioritizing of functions and tasks so that staff time could be focused on projects more consistent with the direction in which the organization needed to move. Two time-consuming "sacred cow" projects were dropped, thus reducing the drain on staff energy. Walter and the consultants also argued for the creation of a new development director position, in order to address the funding problems head-on. Some fearful board members were hesitant because that seemed to denote spending money they didn't have. But the gamble paid off. Within the year, the new development director had brought in three times her salary. Walter, meanwhile, got to hand off the fund-raising to a professional and do what he did best—program development and staff supervision.

A final recommendation of the consultants was a radical attempt to forge a closer working relationship between the board and staff members. They helped to launch a board-staff "buddy system," in which each board member was assigned a staffer to consult with periodically, in order to keep the board informed of the perspectives and concerns of staff, and to facilitate collaboration on procedural improvements and new project development. With new funding coming in, there was, for the first time in several years, the possibility of building rather than cutting. Very quickly the ultimatums and the blaming stopped, and Walter found himself heading up a rejuvenated organization.

And Karen, the controller living in fear of the cost-cutting chief financial officer? Like Walter, Karen decided that she preferred to stay where she was, but that she would leave if the strategy she devised didn't work. The first thing we did was to take a hard look at why the CFO made her so nervous. I asked her what her mother was like. Bingo! "I have to say she's pretty controlling, and also rather secretive," Karen responded to my gentle probes. And so here was a competent adult trying to handle her work challenges while still under the influence of what it had felt like to be a fearful child struggling to please an unpredictable parent.

Once we did some exercises to separate Karen's little-girl feelings about her mother from her reactions to her current boss, she was on her way to dealing more effectively with the CFO. She decided to do some research herself and then approach her boss directly to discuss the merits of additional outsourcing moves. The CFO was surprised (but pleased) with her new forthrightness and agreed to talk. Karen arranged to do extensive benchmarking (researching what similar organizations were doing) and bring back comparison costs to the CFO. Together they hammered out a plan for cutting costs within the current system. Karen's bronchitis didn't need to return, and she found that she had a great deal to learn from her boss now that they had a different kind of relationship.

What about Bernard, the out-of-control school superintendent? Well, Bernard also decided to get some outside help. First, he used the next school vacation not to supervise the installation of a new computer system, as he had planned, but rather to take a week-long stay at a health retreat. There he learned about diet, exercise, yoga, meditation, relationships, and the importance of talking out his frustrations. He came back with a carefully designed regimen for himself and monthly appointments to return for check-ins. He also found that in just a week he had more energy than he had had since taking the job. Then he felt able to step back and take a longer view of his problems.

The next expert he talked to was a managerial competencies consultant, who told him what he already knew about himself—his problems with boundaries, poor attention to detail, and excessive need to please were undercutting his strengths as a coalition builder and program developer. With his consultant's help, Bernard collected feedback from others in the school system about his performance. Together they forged a plan built on that feedback. Bernard delegated some of the tasks he was currently doing, and identified some things that just didn't need to happen anymore, such as detailed monthly reports of meetings, personally handling all parent calls, and visiting each school every week.

He also got school committee approval to promote his most organized, detail-oriented administrative assistant to be an office manager, with responsibility for organizing his calendar, moving work around in the office more efficiently, and generally protecting Bernard from himself.

His next move was to seek some negotiation training for himself through a local conflict-resolution consulting group, to prepare for getting the school committee, administrators, faculty, students, and parents on board to tackle the real culprit—the tax-cut legislation that was driving the funding shortfalls. Bernard's "builder" skills had a mission again. Together, his coalition of teachers, kids, and parents helped to pass an override to the restricted spending legislation and the budget was restored to within 2 percent of former levels.

Does the story have a fairy-tale ending? Did his fiancée return? Sometimes the train *does* pull out just as you're running breathlessly up the platform to catch it. There was no salvaging that relationship, but Bernard figured it might be better for him to have learned that lesson the hard way. He decided to concentrate on his friendships for a while, confident that if he continued to make time for a real life, then someone right for him would come along.

And Rob, the twice-fired software engineer? When he and I sat down to talk, he was already putting the pieces together to see these two false starts as a signal of some kind. "My chiropractor gave me a lecture about how stress and back pain are related," he said. "He asked me to think about what unnecessary loads I was carrying around."

"Any ideas about that?" I asked. It turned out that Rob and his wife Jen had indeed taken the question seriously. After several weeks of soul searching, they had come to a startling conclusion. "It's our house," he said, "our supposed dream house overlooking the ocean. But we're young, with no kids—and we don't really need it. I think we bought it to impress our friends and show our parents we were adults. But we're too stressed out paying for it to enjoy it."

The rest was almost easy, because Rob and Jen had gone to the heart (or perhaps, the back) of the matter. It took only a month to sell the house and find an apartment in the funky neighborhood where they had lived as newlyweds. Jen's income was enough to sustain them in the apartment. Rob, meanwhile, was able to take the profit from the house sale and invest in his own small software-development operation. "I'm an adolescent at heart," he explained, "so I'm really hooked on the idea of 'edutainment.' I hated school because it was so boring. It would feel terrific to create computer learning games for use in schools and youth centers." And that's exactly what he did. When we last talked, his back wasn't hurting and he had just turned a profit for the first time. As for impressing their friends, he reported that most of them were insanely jealous of the freedom and opportunity he had found.

Finally, there's Emily, the rising young whiz with Chronic Fatigue Syndrome. Once we began digging around a little in Emily's life, she blurted out, "I'm just so tired (*hmm*) of doing work that has so little intellectual challenge, and so little time to make real connections to people." Emily considered lots of options for being in a more intellectual environment. Obviously, a college campus would be fun. But she rejected the idea of a Ph.D. and starting out on the tenure-track marathon, because it felt that for her academic life would be in many ways as limiting as publishing. She also figured out that she wanted to work with people on an emotional as well as an intellectual level. After much debate about money, location, and whether it was okay to walk out on an organization that she knew was hoping to push her on up the ladder, Emily put together a three-step plan.

First, she networked with friends and college classmates in communications and in fund-raising, and found a job as a senior development writer at a major West Coast university. Next, she attended as many seminars and workshops as she could on writing therapy—learning methods for helping people with writer's block and for using writing as a therapeutic tool. Armed with a networking list from her college, she did information interviews with both expressive therapists and writing teachers to ask how they had done their training and to test out which approach felt more comfortable to her. At the same time, she also began a series of visits with a body-mind counselor, who helped her lay out a routine of nutrition, exercise, adequate rest, and playful relationships. Within several months, her CFS symptoms had abated.

Now it was time to make some decisions. The course she chose was pursuing a Master of Social Work degree part-time at the university where she worked. She planned then to do one of her fieldwork placements at the university counseling service, where she would be able to use writing as part of her work with students. She also started doing some of her own writing of poetry and short fiction. It felt terrific to be back on a campus again, able to attend lectures, concerts, readings, and exhibits whenever she could carve out the time. It was much cheaper to live in a university town than it had been in New York, and so the cut in pay had negligible results. The reduction in stress, however, had a tremendous payoff. Emily's case is such a critical one because it illustrates how easy it is to let your own successes sweep you along a path you don't really want to be on. As we were finishing our most recent check-in session during one of her visits east, Emily said, "I'm very glad I got the message from my body early on about needing to move out of publishing. What if I had waited ten or fifteen years until I was really saddled with more debt and responsibility?"

And what about you? Does your intuition tell you that things at work can get less toxic with time, or do you need to be sculpting some changes for yourself? Your work dissatisfactions are uniquely your own. They appear at the intersection where the demands imposed on you at work meet your own relentlessly evolving requirements for emotional, intellectual, and spiritual development. What makes work toxic for you is probably quite different from what's creating symptoms for someone else in your work unit.

Still, some general principles apply. For most of us, the world of work we entered is not the one we're in today. Now is the time to take stock of and respond creatively to the following new, inescapable and mostly permanent realities:

- Expect more pressure, greater demands, and fewer people employed on-site to do the work. That's why loving what you do has never been more important—if your work doesn't excite you, the accelerated expectations will be unbearable.
- Cost-cutting will be the official sport of most organizations, both for-profits and nonprofits; budgets will run very close to the wire. For managers, a blend of fiscal skills and creative problem-solving will be required. Everybody else will need to contribute increased adaptability, a good nose for efficiencies of various sorts, and a willingness to join in rather than resist the need to control costs.

- Uncertainty will prevail. The only thing you can count on is your own ability to land on your feet when you get knocked off balance by a shift in policy or practice. If your work unit hasn't made some major changes in how things are done in the past year, watch out: you may be comfortably on a path to extinction.
- Increasingly, work will be done primarily in teams. If you're a middle manager who has gotten used to being a little higher up on the totem pole, prepare for collaborating with direct reports as equals in teams. Your ideas will be judged for their merit, rather than in deference to your position. That shift may surprise you. But don't resist, and try not to take it in the ego.
- Constant learning will be required, particularly in technology. If you've been shying away from numbers or computers, the only useful advice is to find the training or coaching you need to "get over it." There are lots of books, videos, and tutors to show you how. One of the best strategies for breaking the electronic barrier for yourself is to have a computer and some games at home. Learn to *play* on it, and *working* on it will come much more easily.
- You'll need to take responsibility for choreographing your own career and underwriting your own retirement; formerly paternalistic organizations have gotten out of the business of taking care of people. So much for hanging on in a job you don't much like just to get vested in the pension fund. Change that strategy *now*!

In some organizations, managers and human resources professionals are helping people understand and function more effectively in this unfamiliar "post-corporate" environment, with group training sessions and individual coaching. But in other organizations, the people in charge are duplicating mistakes Ellen's boss made, making arbitrary moves and driving out many of their most creative, autonomous, and self-respecting people—the ones they need most. They are scaring off and wearing out their best talent by making hastily conceived and poorly communicated changes, failing to prioritize added tasks, short-cutting the training needed to introduce new practices and mandates, pitting groups of workers against each other, and forgetting to let people know how their work is valued and appreciated.

Perhaps it's poetic justice that the people most likely to knuckle under and stay on in a state of misery are probably the ones organizations need least. People who remain frightened and angry, the passive-aggressive ones, are more likely to suffer and persevere. But those employees will be unable to manage the complex projects that increasingly require creativity, flexibility, and teamwork—because they have become beaten down by anger, distrust, and alienation.

The most important message, however, is not about your boss or your organization—it's about you. For sure, many Americans are feeling abused or betrayed in some way by their work. And many work units are virtual disaster areas in terms of fairness and worker satisfaction. But the only person with the power to turn the *dissatisfactions* and *catastrophes* in your work life into *catalysts* for keeping yourself healthy, and productive, and spiritually alive is you. Only you can choreograph the life you really need to have.

2. Just How Toxic *Is* Your Work?

In order to alter our projections, we must first refocus the projector: we must change ourselves. —KEN DYCHTWALD

Have you tried to measure just how much what's happening at work might be getting to you? Perhaps the Stress Detector below can give you some clues:

STRESS DETECTOR: WHAT'S WORKING ON YOU AT WORK THESE DAYS?

For each of the items below, circle the number which best describes *how often* you have felt the following concerns (1 = almost never, 2 = sometimes, 3 = often, 4 = almost always).

Anxiety

- I'm afraid I won't have enough money.   1 2 3 4
- I'm worried I won't find another job if I lose this one.   1 2 3 4
- I'm worried about having to learn so many new   1 2 3 4
  things.
- I want things to stay the way they've always been.   1 2 3 4
- I worry about what might go wrong in new situa-   1 2 3 4
  tions.
- I have trouble sleeping because I wake up thinking   1 2 3 4
  about what's happening at work.

Anger

- I find myself getting irritable or angry at work.   1 2 3 4
- I find myself getting irritable or angry away from work.   1 2 3 4
- I'm angry about increased demands at work.   1 2 3 4
- I get impatient with other people's mistakes.   1 2 3 4
- I blame particular people for what's happening at work and think about getting even with them.   1 2 3 4
- I find myself speeding impatiently from one task to another.   1 2 3 4

Lack of Control

- I feel I don't have enough say in how my work gets done.   1 2 3 4
- It doesn't seem that my opinion is valued enough at work.   1 2 3 4
- I know I'm ready for more challenge and responsibility, but I just can't get it in my current job.   1 2 3 4
- I have so much work that it's impossible to do it all well.   1 2 3 4
- I don't feel that I'm appreciated or trusted enough.   1 2 3 4
- It's unnerving that the people in charge don't really know what they're doing.   1 2 3 4

Lack of Confidence

- I wonder whether I'm really doing a good enough job.   1 2 3 4
- I worry about what others think of me.   1 2 3 4
- I'm afraid that people will discover my shortcomings.   1 2 3 4
- I'm worried that I won't be able to keep up with what's expected of me as the demands increase.   1 2 3 4
- I'm afraid that my reputation at work will keep me from getting the assignments and promotions I would like.   1 2 3 4
- I'm afraid I'm not really capable of doing a great job.   1 2 3 4

Shut-Down Feelings

- I have trouble knowing what I'm really feeling.   1 2 3 4
- It doesn't seem safe to express what I'm feeling   1 2 3 4
  at home.
- It seems that nobody at work wants to know what   1 2 3 4
  I'm feeling.
- I hold my feelings in until they finally erupt in some   1 2 3 4
  way.
- Nobody really understands how I feel about things.   1 2 3 4
- I don't really trust feelings.   1 2 3 4

Diminished Relationships

- I spend lots of time alone.   1 2 3 4
- It's hard to make enough time for family and friends.   1 2 3 4
- People close to me complain that I'm not available   1 2 3 4
  enough.
- It's hard for me to get close to people.   1 2 3 4
- I seem to end up arguing with people more than   1 2 3 4
  I'd like.
- I'm too worn out to give much time to relationships.   1 2 3 4

Few people have scores entirely to the right or left on the grid; most find that their numbers snake across the page, revealing an interesting scatter of stressors. One of the difficulties with negative emotions is that they tend to run together into one dark clump, making it hard to know what really has you on edge. The Stress Detector grid lets you pull them apart to see more clearly the pattern of your own reactions to what's happening in your life.

Take the time to review the statements where you've circled twos, threes, and fours. Then share your responses with someone you trust. If your responses fall more to the right-hand side of the numbers, chances are your stress quotient is high, and you need to be talking about it. If your confidant is a co-worker, that person will benefit from the discussion too, so long as you focus on problem-solving rather than on "ain't it awful" stories.

Indeed, stressors do cause physiological reactions. When you feel stressed, for instance, your brain stimulates your kidneys to secrete hormones that prepare you to defend yourself, sending increased levels of fats, cholesterol, and sugar into your bloodstream. The immune system is depressed during such reactions, lowering your ability to combat diseases. Concurrently, adrenaline-related substances are at work, increasing your heart rate and constricting your arteries to prepare you for battle. The alarm has been sounded, and you're ready.

In the case of ongoing work stress, after a while this combat alert begins to take its toll. The greater the stress reaction, the more likely it is that your body will be strained. Prolonged high levels of cholesterol, blood pressure, and heart rate tax the cardiovascular system. As cardiologist Dean Ornish explains, "Emotional stress profoundly increases the occurrence of sudden cardiac death via a series of interactions between the brain and the heart."[1] The diminished immune reaction, meanwhile, leaves you more vulnerable to all kinds of infections.

So let's take a closer look at your "score" on the Stress Detector: each one of these six factors has been shown by extensive medical research to correlate with major health problems. When events on the job create these reactions, then your work is in danger of becoming toxic. For each of the six stressors in this chapter, you'll find body-mind research documenting why it's harmful, as well as practical suggestions for managing it. As we saw with the psychological hardiness research, stressors themselves don't necessarily engender stress and illness. People have to help the process along.

Anxiety: When You Can't Stop Thinking About It

One thing you can own free and clear in this world is your interpretation of it. —Deepak Chopra

Anxiety stems from worrying unnecessarily about what might be coming next. When that sense of uncertainty is prolonged and turns into chronic stress, you become more prone to cardiovascular illness. You also lose your ability to fight off diseases of various kinds. In a thirteen-year study of four thousand patients from the Centers for Disease Control in Atlanta, people who experienced their lives as stressful were twice as likely to develop ulcers as those who didn't.[2]

The number one killer of Americans is coronary heart disease, accounting for half of all U.S. deaths. Coronary heart disease is twice as prevalent as all forms of cancer combined. One of the most significant causes of heart disease is anxiety. For most employed Americans, the primary source of anxiety is work, thanks in large part to diminishing job security and increasing workloads. Impending changes prowl the hallways of most organizations these days, it seems, ready to pounce on unprotected workers. Chronic worry that comes from perceived vulnerability has also been blamed for susceptibility to infections and impaired memory. And it has been implicated in a variety of other medical problems, ranging in scope from poor concentration to irritability, sleep disturbance, muscle tension, nausea, dizziness, difficulty in swallowing, loose bowel movements, fluctuations in weight, and even increased dental cavities. In one study combining the findings from 101 other studies, people who were chronically worried, sad, or mad had double the risk of disease.

If you scored high on the anxiety section of the quiz, you probably know firsthand that anxious thoughts have a way of begetting more anxious thoughts, particularly in the middle of the night, when they often come calling. So it's critical to be able to confront the irrational thought processes that spawn anxieties by asking yourself a few questions. The next time fear creeps up on you, try writing down your responses to these four queries:

Anti-Anxiety Review

- What is the worst thing that could happen?
- How likely is it that this terrible thing will in fact occur?
- If it did happen, how would I handle it? What people could I call on to help me?

- What record of successes in other difficult situations do I have to draw on as evidence that I'll be able to handle whatever comes along?

(Put most of your energy into the last question—don't give up until you have at least several good answers. Once you do, you'll very likely feel the anxiety slither back down inside you.)

In the past, you've handled situations you had previously never dreamed you could. And even though it's hard to remember them when irrational fear taps you on the shoulder, you will handle them again. Some people do have bona fide anxiety attacks that can't be quelled without medical interventions. A conversation with your health-care practitioner, a counselor, or the Employee Assistance Program specialist where you work can help you decide whether you're someone who would benefit from professional help. Most people, however, can learn to massage their own thought processes to stay out of the grip of anxiety, boldly reassuring themselves, "I'll handle it."

Jim learned to manage his anxieties during his first six months in a corporate training program, where eighty-hour weeks and impossible assignments were just part of the drill. At my suggestion, he found another member of the group who seemed as anxious about "flunking out" as he was, and they learned to zip through the Anti-Anxiety Review questions together as a major presentation or interview approached. Each one had identified a list of successes to call up and share with the other when anxiety threatened. For Jim, it was a strange combination: becoming an eagle scout, getting his first varsity letter, opening the letter saying he was a National Merit Semifinalist, and playing the comic lead in a play his sophomore year in college. In each of these situations, he had fretted and fretted about the possibility of failing or making a fool of himself—but things had turned out fine. The "program" we devised worked for him because he was willing to superimpose these successes on whatever doubts sneaked in during high-demand times.

Fortunately, your body can help too. One of the most effective antidotes is something you have with you all the time—your lungs. You can interrupt the progression of anxious thoughts by taking deep diaphragmatic breaths and instructing your mind to be still. When you breathe like a very young child, pulling air deep into the bottom of your lungs, feeling your belly expand, you pump added oxygen into your bloodstream. That's because most of the alveoli, or small, capillary-rich sacs where the exchange of oxygen and carbon dioxide takes place, are located at the bottom of your lungs. When you take shallow breaths, which you do especially when you're afraid, the alveoli can't do their work, and so you don't send your "highest octane" blood out to fuel your body.

Breathing deeply, on the other hand, sends well-oxygenated blood out to your brain and other organs, making them able to function much more effectively. Sitting quietly with your eyes closed, concentrating only on slow, deep breathing for two minutes or so, can add a physiological boost to your efforts at reality-checking. The calming effect is truly amazing.

Jon Kabat-Zinn, director of the Stress Reduction Clinic at the University of Massachusetts Medical Center, teaches his students of "mindfulness" that dealing successfully with anxiety requires you to slow down all your activities, deliberately inserting meditative pauses whenever possible into your work schedule. He also suggests simple things like changing into casual clothes as soon as you get home and not thinking about work in the evening as you recuperate from the stresses of the day.[3] That may seem hard, but the harder it seems, the more you probably need to do it.

Anger: When You're Mad More Than You Want to Be

Those of us who are locked into ineffective expressions of anger suffer as deeply as those of us who dare not get angry at all.   —Harriet Lerner

Hostility is another primary cause of coronary heart disease. In the 1960s, more than five thousand University of North Carolina undergraduates took the Minnesota Multiphasic Personality Inventory, a standard psychological assessment tool. Researchers assigned each of the subjects a hostility score, based on the results of the MMPI, and then for the next several decades tracked the course of their health records. The results were sobering. The more hostile subjects were consistently more likely to smoke, weighed more, drank more, and had higher levels of cholesterol.[4] In a more recent Harvard Medical School study, researchers found that anger doubled the risk of heart attack for people with pre-existing heart disease.[5] A tendency to get mad about what's happening at work is clearly not a health-enhancer.

"Angry? Of course I'm angry," Carl snapped at me as we talked about how things were going at the hospital where he was a nurse. "I've worked every damned shift they've asked me to for five years now, giving up weekends and holidays with barely any notice at all sometimes, just to stay on the good side of the nursing supervisor. And what do I get for that? Because our unit's not profitable enough any longer, they're closing us down. What else could I be but mad?"

Some people, like Carl, are angry about the changes happening in organizations because they seem like a personal affront. "My company used to care about me and now I'm just a cost to be cut," they say. This is particularly true for people who once felt a strong loyalty to their employer. Their anger is problematic not only for them, but also for co-workers caught in the cross-fire. When people all around you are angry, you have some choices about how to respond to them. You can, of course, get caught up in the generally acrid environment their anger creates, yelling back at them or allowing your feelings to get hurt. Or you can practice some strategies for consciously distancing from the toxicity, by rearranging how your work gets done or by mental gymnastics such as imagining the angry person being farther and farther away from you or having a voice so low it can't be heard. You have everything to gain by staying out of range, physically or psychologically.

For other people—labeled Type A's by some psychologists—anger is not situational but generally part of their speedy, impatient, often hostile style. Type A's were in trouble before downsizing speeded up the merry-go-round and piled on work, but now many of them are seemingly crazed, going faster and faster, and filling their organizations with demanding and disapproving vibrations. It's obvious that this creates a toxic environment for their co-workers, subordinates, and supervisors. What is less obvious, however, is how frequent anger harms the person who's feeling it. Study after study shows that staying chronically angry predisposes you to a wide range of illnesses.

But what can you do about your own anger, whether you're a lifelong impatient type or now find yourself being chronically cranky in a hard-to-take situation? If you're working in a place that makes you angry now and didn't before, something must have changed: your boss, your co-workers, the demands, the rules? You must figure out whether it would be safe (1) to express your frustrations and (2) to try to make some further course-corrections in what's going on. So why not discuss those options with a trustworthy person or two? You may figure out a way to open the release valve on some of your own anger and get some improvements percolating at work.

If you and your confidants conclude that the stressors themselves are not likely to be changed at work, then you have two options—to change your job or to change yourself. Changing your job could be accomplished in a number of ways. Finding a new one is certainly possible. But you don't always have to leave to get a change. Switching assignments, working on another team, or making other kinds of adjustments can mitigate anger. Jill, for instance, discovered that meeting with one of the unit heads with whom her department often collaborated made her angry because his militaristic style reminded her so much of her father. So she asked her assistant manager, who didn't mind "the captain's" style so much, if she wanted to take on the additional responsibility of being the liaison to that department. It was a win-win. The assistant got a career boost and Jill didn't get a migraine every Tuesday at nine a.m. at the project meeting.

Jill was smart enough, however, to know that this was not the only overbearing colleague she was going to meet in her career. So she went one step further and made an appointment with the counselor at her HMO, to talk about how she might learn to handle people who "pushed her buttons." After ten sessions of brief cognitive therapy, exploring and deciding to put aside the negative interpretations she brought to certain situations, she felt much less likely to get angry at overly pushy types. Some people are able to use friends and partners, support groups, or even self-help groups to take the sting out of work situations that make them angry again and again. Whether you do it by yourself, with the help of friends, or with professional help, don't let anger be your constant companion. The price is just too high.

Lack of Control: When Your Life Is Running Away with You

No society can grow healthy individuals if it does not foster personal hope, optimism, commitment, and self-worth.
—WILLIAM POOLE

People sense a loss of control in a variety of ways. Such disparate problems as too much work, too little opportunity to manage your own assignments, too little freedom of movement, lack of career mobility, lack of respect from others for the abilities you know you have, and feeling you can't make any progress financially all contribute to a pervasive sense of powerlessness. That felt impotence on your part soon translates into emotional and physical symptoms.

One sure way to make people sick is to ask them to do more and more work and then give them little or no control over how it gets done. That's what researchers in the now-famous Framingham Heart Study found: the people most likely to have heart disease were those whose jobs levied high demands with very little autonomy.[6]

A Swedish study shed some light on the physical effects of control when it compared the reactions of commuters on a morning train ride. Researchers found that riders who boarded the train seventy-nine minutes from Stockholm experienced much less stress, as measured by increases in their adrenaline levels, than commuters who had only a forty-three-minute ride. How could this be? How could a longer ride be less stressful than a shorter one?

The research team concluded that, because the group who boarded earlier entered an empty train, they had many more opportunities to exercise control over where and with whom they sat, as well as over how to arrange their carry-ons. Meanwhile, commuters who boarded a crowded train farther down the line experienced much less choice and control over their destiny.[7] When you feel that you have some control over how your work gets done, you are much less likely to experience stress and illness, no matter how challenging the assignments might be.

Yet another factor making people feel out of control at work is the absence of opportunity for advancement. "No place to go" is a complaint I hear frequently, particularly in organizations where both resources and middle management advancement options have dried up. At mighty IBM, for instance, half of the workforce has been downsized in the past decade; that leaves much less room for moving around in the organization. Employees who for one reason or another can't leave often find themselves feeling terribly stuck, another situation fraught with physical and emotional risk.

Another phenomenon pushing people into feeling out of control is the sense of moving backward rather than forward financially, as working harder seems to beget only more bills. Newspaper and magazine articles scream at us about the bankruptcy of the Medicare and Social Security systems and the destitution awaiting us if we don't save more for retirement, when we're already limping from paycheck to paycheck. Against the backdrop of record-level corporate profits and escalating compensation for senior management, working harder for not enough money is doubly hard to take.

If having more discretionary money would help you feel more in control, there are many ways to accomplish that. Start with spending less for things that *don't* give you the sense of security and control you're seeking—that involves "checking in with yourself" to ask some questions about those feelings. There are many good books on the subject of being thrifty and stretching your resources. One of my favorites, *Your Money or Your Life*, by Joe Dominguez and Vicki Robin, addresses very well the sticky problems of staying solvent and keeping your spending congruent with your major values. Both are important to your sense of control.

Or you could make more. You could work outside the system to develop your revenue-generating capabilities. Starting a small business or service venture on your own time, free-lancing your talents as a writer, photographer, designer, or artist, or massaging connections in your industry to use should you decide to sell your talents "outside" as a consultant are all possible strategies. Launching your own venture on the side can be tiring, but many people find the autonomy therapeutic. If you want to go for more money inside your organization, a good way to start would be talking to your manager or to someone in human resources, depending on the politics of your organization, about what you'd need to do to be ready for a raise or a promotion. Sometimes, positioning yourself to demand more money happens by getting a better offer somewhere else and parlaying that into a promotion or a raise in your current spot. Whatever approach feels right, you must take control—sitting around hoping to be recognized and rewarded just won't do.

Lack of control is often harder to fix than anxiety or anger, because you can't just wrest authority away from the people in charge. Over the past several years, however, people have shared with me the strategies (some subtle, some bolder) that they've used to feel more in control of things at work. One accountant started a lunchtime support group for single mothers in her company and found role-playing with her group helped her to be much more able to negotiate with her manager about flexible time when the children were sick. A government worker took courses in various software applications and got to be the expert in her unit. Soon her job included a role as departmental trouble-shooter, which gave her a feeling that she had designed at least a part of the job to her liking.

Some people opted for direct relief. A small group of union members in a manufacturing facility convinced the union leadership to bargain for optional reduced-rate access to a fitness facility for their members. They released the stress they were carrying around in their bodies by working out on the Cybex machines for half an hour three times a week after work.

A university administrator figured a way to feel more in control of things by joining the university's employee grievance committee. He made some new friends and learned a lot about the workings of the university in general, knowledge which he was then able to use in doing his own work more autonomously and getting his department's projects through the hierarchy. A financial analyst in search of more control negotiated with his manager during his annual performance review to do some cross-training with the marketing department; this gave him more expertise, which he was able to parlay into assignments with more latitude in making decisions.

If you want it, you can have more control at work. First you have to ask yourself if you're willing to take on the responsibility which that entails. If the answer is yes, then you need to strategize about how to do it. Among the strategies I've seen people employ are setting new performance goals with their manager and asking for the training they'll need to meet them; volunteering for new projects that the boss wants done well and negotiating for the desired amount of autonomy; and suggesting task forces and work teams to get jobs done more collaboratively. The possibilities are many. The first step is identifying your particular problem.

Yet another way in which some people allow themselves to be out of control is by neglecting their boundaries and their organizational skills, and feeling overwhelmed much of the time. Many times I ask exhausted clients, "If you could get your work finished in a reasonable amount of time, would you be feeling a need to leave your job now?" Sometimes the answer is yes—people do get tired of doing the same thing or being with the same people. But at other times I get a different response. Bonnie, for instance, was a manager for the Postal Service who had come in saying that she was "drowning" in her current position. When I asked her the question about whether it was the nature or the volume of her work, she stopped short.

"Well, actually, I guess I like what I do," she said, with a look of surprise. "What I can't stand is ending the workday feeling absolutely buried in paperwork and unanswered telephone-call slips. There isn't much on my desk I don't want to do—there just doesn't seem to be enough time to do it."

Like most bad situations, this one had evolved in a variety of ways. The most obvious contributor was indeed the organization. But some of the problems were of Bonnie's making. Because of her lack of boundaries, which kept her from protecting her own time, Bonnie invited co-workers to stop in to share their problems and eat up precious time every day. She also had notoriously poor organizational skills, so that papers were piled up around her work area. She usually met deadlines and kept the work flowing, but almost always in a "running to catch up" mode. Her feelings of frustration, as well as the flu that had returned repeatedly this winter, were telling her that something had to change. On the surface, a new job away from all these piles seemed like the answer. In reality, however, the challenge was Bonnie's.

Bonnie was in luck, because the Postal Service had quite a few efficiency/operations experts around at the time, and so she was able to avail herself of some very helpful consultations about managing time and paper. She also got permission to attend several seminars on topics such as "Setting Limits," "Staying Sane by Saying No," and "Finding the Help You Need." Bonnie came to realize that she had been sabotaging herself for a long time, giving away her time, letting sloppy habits rob her of the sense of control she needed to feel good about her work. She also decided to redesign the functions of the two administrative assistants in the office, to get the help she needed. One of them was a card-carrying efficiency freak who had been hankering for some time to "organize" her boss. Bonnie invited her input, and gave her the assignment to get things flowing smoothly. And she did, much to everyone's relief. If you're someone whose work life seems out of control, seemingly because of pressures at work, you might want to ask yourself to what degree your own work habits might be part of the problem.

But here's the important thing. All of these autonomy-seekers had to propose the changes themselves. You could probably have more control at work too. Why not think about your own situation, and then talk about it with a few well-chosen people? The only thing not to do is to sit by feeling controlled or out of control, eroding your mental and physical health in the process.

Lack of Confidence: When You're Not Sure You Can Do It

Of all the liars in the world, sometimes the worst are your own fears. —RUDYARD KIPLING

Unfortunately, many people begin their working lives already saddled by self-doubt and an inability to trust their successes. But when organizations make it so very clear that they value people less than the bottom line, and keep employees in a constant state of uncertainty, it's even harder for workers to sustain their sense of self-worth. Employees who put a low value on themselves are much more likely to feel unequal to the tasks at hand, and hence much more prone to feelings of helplessness.

The famous Harvard Study of Adult Development, which followed Harvard men from the classes of 1939–44 throughout their adulthood, has provided unequivocal evidence of the health-sustaining power of confidence and optimism. Among this group of hundreds of successful, healthy young men, one of the primary determinants of which ones were able to maintain their health and be successful well into adulthood was a general expectation that things would go well. In myriad studies since then, lowered resistance to infection and chronic conditions such as arthritis and asthma have been shown to be linked to lack of confidence and negative expectations.[8]

Melinda was afraid she would lose her job as a loan officer with a recently acquired savings bank. Because she had been reading a book about body-mind health issues, she had already begun to suspect that her headaches and her recurrent herpes outbreaks might be related to the way in which she was responding to the changes associated with the merger.

"Every time somebody from the new corporate headquarters came down here, supposedly to update us on how our office was going to fit into their plans, they did it in ways that made us feel unnecessary and unwanted," Melinda reported. "Pretty soon I began to wonder if there wasn't something wrong with me. I also found that I was making stupid mistakes whenever they were around."

"And what about your headaches and cold sores? Was there any pattern to them?" I asked. Indeed there was. Melinda realized that the headaches seemed to come just before the scheduled visitations, as she braced herself for the coolness and the suspicion she knew would be forthcoming. The herpes lesions, however, usually popped out several days after the visits, as Melinda reflected on the interaction and fretted about whether she was good enough to be hired anyplace else should the new parent bank decide to close their office. "When I came to work here I seemed to have more confidence," she said quietly. "But somehow I just lost it, and I didn't even know it until it was gone."

For Melinda and perhaps for you, diminished confidence is itself a stressor that turns into a health hazard by keeping you in a state of constant low-level fear. Many physical problems have been linked to the pervasive, ongoing stress of feeling unequal to what you have to do.

Like anger and anxiety, consistently devaluing your accomplishments and expecting to disappoint people can grow out of problematic early-family scripts, or can be a response to the kinds of toxic work environments we've been discussing. Or both. Counseling sessions to help differentiate early family hot spots from current work factors, such as a militaristic boss or impossible demands, are always helpful. If that's possible now, I'd recommend it. But there are also many things you can do on your own.

The first is to acknowledge how much lack of confidence may be undercutting your performance and making you susceptible to illness. The second is to decide to beat it, much as you would a problem with alcohol, food, drugs, or spending. If you really want to stop devaluing yourself, you can.[9] Probably the three most important words for confidence control are "*check it out.*" You can simply ask trusted people questions about what they're experiencing in your presence, or how they think you're doing on a given task, and then you can adjust your self-assessments accordingly. People who take the time to check out their negative perceptions are usually happily surprised at the discrepancy between what they feared and what's real.

If your self-doubt seems to be the hard-to-shake variety, you'll need a longer-term solution. Were you trying to lick a substance-abuse problem, you'd need to pay attention to it every day. You'd make a commitment one day at a time to stay clean, by staying aware of your own feelings and asking for extra strength when you felt tempted to break the contract with yourself. When I'm working with someone on self-doubt, I'll suggest choosing a period of time for immersion in the process—usually three to four weeks. Most experts on habit reformation say that twenty-one consecutive days of a new behavior can be enough to get it well established.

The assignment then is to keep a small notebook labeled "doubter's diary," and carry it in a pocket, purse, or briefcase at all times. For the duration of the process, whenever the old "I'm not good enough" attitude pokes its gloomy head into an otherwise reasonable, happy day, force yourself to stop what you're doing and make these notes in your log:

1. Date, time, and content of the thought
2. What was going on when that doubt overtook you?
3. What prior times did this situation recall for you? (The earlier the better, even back to childhood or adolescence)

4. What successes can you recall to neutralize the doubt you're having now?

5. Are you willing now to let go of the doubt and get on with your day?

If the answer to the last question is yes, visualize yourself scooping up the doubting thoughts and dumping them into the trash. Shake your hands a few times to be rid of the negative energy, and get on with what you were doing. If you're unable at first to say yes to distancing from the doubt at first, stick with it until you can. You might also consider asking yourself whether the correct helping verb is "can't" or "won't." Stubbornness is often a quality of self-doubters: if you're not ready to kick that gruesome habit, nobody else can do it for you.

Frequently people say in sessions, "I just don't have much confidence in myself, you know," as if we should stop and have a moment of silence about it because it's such a tragedy, and nothing can be done about it. Well, it is tragic, actually, but it's a situation where action, not passivity, is required. Self-doubt is incredibly wasteful—it limits your productivity, keeps you from trying new things, and it makes you sick. But only you can decide that you're tired enough of throwing away time, money, opportunity, and happiness to do something about it.

One of the things that helps the doubter's diary work is that it's really inconvenient to stop and answer all those questions. If you do it religiously at first and get a handle on what situations or people are likely to trigger self-doubt for you, then you can strategize about avoiding them or handling them differently. Then, after awhile, you can just zip through the questions in your head and get to the "drop it in the trash" part of the exercise. It is, after all, your resolve to deep-six those self-defeating, self-enervating doubts that matters. The greater your resolve, the shorter your period of remaining enslavement will be.

Some work environments are affirming. Supervisors encourage you to set goals that stretch you but are achievable, and then reward you for attaining them. That kind of management is a lot like good parenting. Self-doubt is less often a problem in those situations. If, however, you find yourself in either a gloomy or very competitive place that feels unsafe at some level, you're more likely to be visited by doubt. But once again the action is with you: as Eleanor Roosevelt said, no one can make you feel inadequate without your permission. So remember to try one of the following proven antidotes:

- Check it out to see if the news is as bad as you think it is. (It seldom is.)
- Ask people who value you for positive feedback to sustain you, so long as you promise to believe them.
- Make your goals more realistic. Just a little reach is all you need. Low-confidence people have a habit of trying to accomplish the impossible.
- Praise yourself when you do something well. Try it—the words won't really choke you. It just seems that way.
- Keep a doubter's diary. You won't be sorry.

Shut-Down Feelings:
When You Don't Feel Much Anymore

Who are you depressed at?   —Fritz Perls

The body-mind literature says in many different ways that closing yourself off from your feelings, either because you learned it in the family or the rules at work require it, is dangerous to your health. One study by David Shapiro, psychiatrist, and Ann Futterman, then a Ph.D. candidate at UCLA, used actors to test whether expressing strong feelings had any effect on the immune system. In the study, actors played intensely emotional scenes, some sad and some joyful, after which their peripheral blood was tested for natural killer cells (infection-fighting immune substances). The tests showed that intensely expressing either negative or positive emotions had markedly enhanced their immune functioning within twenty minutes.[10]

Psychologist Margaret Kemeny, who did her postdoctoral work in immunology at UCLA, chose a traumatic situation to demonstrate that how you express emotions may be critical to your health. In her work with survivors of the 1989 San Francisco earthquake, she also administered tests of subjects' peripheral immune function. In that incredibly stressful situation, the people who were releasing their emotions were producing elevated amounts of infection-fighting immune cells, hence making them less susceptible to disease. She found that feeling and expressing strong emotions, either positive or negative in nature, make us better equipped to resist illness.

She went on to discover, however, that when strong feelings are prolonged, without a break in mood, they tend to deplete the immune system, and thus be maladaptive. The trick is to have a natural flow of emotions, both positive and negative, with natural highs, lows, and regenerative rest stops in between.[11]

Some people may not know what to do with their emotions. *Somatizer* is the name given to a person who generally lacks the ability to express his feelings of distress in words, but instead reveals them through illness. As Nicholas Cummings, former president of the American Psychological Association, observed, "Like energy in physics, the stress caused by emotional conflicts cannot be destroyed, but it can be transformed; and somatizers translate it into physical symptoms that are easier for them to acknowledge than the psychological issues."[12] People who seem uncomfortable with feelings or who have trouble knowing or expressing what's really going on for them internally seem to be particularly at risk for skin problems. Harvard psychologist Ted Grossbart suggests that people should be "helped to feel the hurt in their hearts rather than in their skin."[13]

But that's not the only danger in repressing emotions. In studies of patients with malignant melanoma, psychologists in San Francisco found a tendency to strong physical reactions to a mild electrical shock, but an unwillingness to talk about it. They coined the term *Type C personality* to describe people who are uncomplaining, cooperative, resistant to expressing negative emotions— and more likely to get cancer.[14]

But what's the alternative to shutting down, in a work culture that seems so uncomfortable with emotion? Obviously, experiences in your "first family" very likely have a great deal to do with your own proclivity to put a lid on your feelings. Perhaps it was to get approval that you learned not to express feelings. Or maybe you saw too much emotion around you and decided to avoid it to stay safe. The people laying out the NO FEELINGS HERE signs at work undoubtedly have their own family story to tell. No matter what the cause of your current state of distancing from your emotions, however, the task of the moment is to reconnect. As Daniel Goleman pointed out in *Emotional Intelligence*, "emotionally tone deaf" people are problematic for themselves, their families, and organization.[15]

You might start with one safe person, either at home or at work, and talk about the questions below. If you're really separated from your feelings much of the time, you might try asking the "feelings coach" you've chosen to let you know when you seem to be in the throes of some strong emotion, as evidenced by your facial expression or body language. It's amazing how often people around you know you're mad or sad before you do. Once you or somebody else has realized you have some emotions swimming up to the surface, ask yourself these questions:

- What feelings are you having?
- When have you had them before?
- What has made these feelings seem unsafe—both now and when you were a child?
- What would you need to make it safe to feel those feelings?

Perhaps you'll want a hug, even permission to cry, or somebody's approval for feeling whatever emotion you've uncovered. Some people keep a lid on their feelings because they're afraid of crying. Researchers at the Dry Eye and Tear Research Center in Minnesota, however, have found that crying is actually a very healthy thing to do. Not only does it make you feel better emotionally, but, because tears contain stress hormones, crying lets you excrete stress chemicals that undercut your health.[16]

When what you're feeling is tamped down, shut off, those feelings you're not wanting to bring to the surface writhe around inside you and compromise your well-being and health. If your responses to the "shut-down feelings" section in this quiz showed you that you've disconnected from your feelings, to stay employed or to survive difficult work relationships, you may be keeping the peace at your own physical peril.

Diminished Relationships:
When There's Not Much Joy in Connecting

Compulsive overworking is the only lifeboat guaranteed to sink. —BRYAN ROBINSON

An unfortunate outcome of being disconnected from your feelings is the attendant difficulty in making connections to other people. Perhaps you see some evidence of that in your stress profile. Whether your relationships are diminished in number or quality, the effect is detrimental to your health. Keeping relationships vital takes time and energy, and there's not much of either to spare in a work-dominated life. When the demands of your job, and how you respond to them, undercut the quality of your family life and friendships, you are robbed of the very things you need in order to be fully alive, and hence most creative and productive on the job.

People who are lonely, struggling in unhappy relationships, or divorced are at greater risk for heart disease, cancer, and a range of chronic conditions. When sociologists reviewed data from a series of large, controlled studies, they found that limited or stressful social relationships were equal to smoking, high blood pressure, high blood cholesterol, obesity, and physical inactivity as risk factors for illness and early death.[17]

Myra was thirty-eight and single, and had just gotten a major promotion to partner at the architectural firm where she worked. She was making more money than she had ever dreamed possible. So why was she feeling so terrible, fighting alternating bouts of colitis and allergies? Demands at the office kept escalating: every surface in her office and her condo was filled with partially completed projects. So how could she be expected to make more time for her friends, when every time she went out, she felt incredibly guilty about the piles she left behind? Having people over was impossible—it would take too long to get things organized and cleaned up, even if she could spare the few hours to cook and entertain.

For a while, her friends and family were understanding, but then Myra began to hear the anger in their voices as she put them off again and again, choosing to stay at home amidst the mess, inhaling junk food and obsessing about why she was so tired and irritable. "I feel as if my wheels are spinning on a muddy road," she said, "and I'm sinking in deeper all the time."

She was pretty surprised the next Sunday morning when four of her friends rang her doorbell and marched in, announcing that they had brought a healthy take-out brunch and were there to help organize the piles. At first she was panicked: what if they got one of her projects messed up? Her best friend Deb saw the look on her face and came over, arms outstretched, to give her a hug. "We're here to help, you know," she said. "You might as well relax and show us what to do."

Myra did, and miraculously, the five old friends spent a productive and hilarious Sunday. "There's a price for this, you know," Deb said as they were leaving. "You must promise *not* to work on Friday or Saturday nights, and you have to do something with other people at least one night of every weekend—or we'll harass you unmercifully. We're not going to stand by and let you make yourself seriously sick. Is it a deal?"

Myra knew they were right, but she felt caught between gratitude for having such wonderful friends and panic about not having enough time to meet her obligations. For a moment, she was paralyzed. Four people peered at her intently, waiting for the words that took so long to form. Finally, she was able to say, "It's a deal."

It wasn't easy for Myra to follow through on that commitment, but having the piles organized, prioritized, and in some cases, delegated, did help. Whenever Friday night came and she felt an urge to fall into the comfortable rut of "just working on some plans for a little while," she picked up the phone and called one of the energetic foursome to whom she had made the promise. After a month of "forced" socializing on weekends, Myra found that she had more energy—and many fewer piles around her dining room. "Friendships are pretty potent medicine," she said. "Somebody ought to bottle it." The irony she had discovered—that you can be more efficient and focused when you take the time to nurture your relationships—is also an essential component of good health.

All of us have our own emotional rhythms. Relationships have a natural ebb and flow, even when work isn't getting in the way. So a somewhat depressed score on the relationships section of the stress quiz may or may not be reflecting major problems. Almost all relationships can be reclaimed, if you're willing to be both honest and gentle, and if you really want the relationship to be vital again. It's important to work toward unveiling and resolving conflicts—not brutally, but respectfully. Myra's friends, for instance, had decided to give her one more chance to come around before telling her how discounted they felt when she ignored them.

Family therapists often tell their clients, "Go have a good fight, so we can talk about it next week." The ground rules for a "good fight" are:

- Really listen to the other person, without formulating your defense while the other is talking.
- Don't generalize; that is, don't say such things as "You always . . ." or "You never. . . ."
- Talk about how it makes you feel, not about the merits of the case: the merits are debatable; how you feel isn't.

Good arguments, by the way, almost always leave people who are trying hard to understand each other feeling closer than before.

Whether you're trying to breathe more vitality into your friendships, build better relationships with your family, or revive a sexual partnership, the elements are the same. You must do all of the following:

- Tune in to your feelings and express them as honestly as possible.
- Care about the relationship.
- Fight vigorously but fairly when necessary.
- Find the humor in it all.

If you do, you'll be a lot healthier for the effort.

Even If Nobody Else Is Listening, Your Body Is

Illness is a negative feedback system. It tells us what we need to stop doing. —CARL O. SIMONTON

There's a story told at Findhorn, the internationally known spiritual center in Scotland, about a man who had just arrived at a spiritual school where he was about to begin his studies. As he left his room, he noticed a mop and bucket sitting in a corner in the hallway. It crossed his mind that it seemed out of place—someone was not taking care of details and putting things away. Each time he went past that spot, he saw the mop and the bucket, and became increasingly annoyed. "You'd think they'd take better care of the place," he muttered to himself. It didn't dawn on him for a while that each time he passed, the mop and bucket were a little farther away from the corner, until he came by one day and found the bucket dead center in the hall. He finally got the message that they were meant for him; one of his spiritual lessons was that he needed to notice what was to be done—such as cleaning the floor. Likewise, when something in your life needs attention, you'd best not try to hurry on by. There's simply no escaping it for very long. Whatever you try to avoid, about your work or other parts of your life, will inevitably show up in a symptom of some kind.

The interactive nature of external events, and your emotional and physical reactions to them, can make work toxic. Body-mind research, which has flourished in the past decade, shows that, though you may try to keep what you're thinking and feeling under wraps, your body knows everything that's going on. There simply are no internal secrets. When you feel distressed, or undervalued, or overwhelmed at work, or when you expect things to go badly, your body responds in a variety of ways.

Certainly, not all illness is caused by career stress. Some people who love their work get sick, and some people whose careers aren't going so well stay healthy. On average, however, people with jobs that are satisfying to them are more likely to stay healthy than those who have chosen work that doesn't fit or who are working in toxic organizations. Many studies have documented the relationship between work stress and health problems, including research with twin siblings of men who had heart disease: in case after case, what separated the healthy from the unhealthy twin was the degree of work satisfaction each one had experienced.[18] Clearly, your mind writes the program that your body dutifully follows. Acknowledging that connection has been one of the major intellectual breakthroughs of this century.

Like many discoveries, the story of the body-mind relationship came together through a series of mistakes, or situations in which the researchers thought at first they must be doing something wrong. In 1974, Robert Ader, a psychologist at the University of Rochester School of Medicine, was involved in a classic conditioning experiment, teaching white rats to reject saccharine-flavored water by pairing it with a nausea-producing drug. Once the rats paired the taste of the saccharine with the nausea-inducing effects of the experimental drug, they would be "conditioned" to associate nausea with the taste of saccharine, even after the nausea drug was no longer being administered.

Ader was puzzled, however, when the young and previously healthy rats began to die, for no apparent reason. So he did further research into the nausea-producing drug and discovered that it also had immune-suppressing effects. Therefore, as the rats imbibed the water that was sweetened (but no longer laced with the nausea-producing drug), not only did their "conditioned" brains tell them to be nauseated without the drug, but their "conditioned" immune systems had also "learned" to be less effective. And so they eventually succumbed to the attacks of the assorted "invaders" from which normally vigilant immune systems protect animals of all species.

Ader was stunned. This could not be happening if the brain and immune system were separate entities. Had he discovered that the immune system could be influenced by what an organism "believed"? He consulted with immunologist Nicholas Cohen at the University of Rochester, and together they launched the effort that has culminated in an avalanche of research about the body-mind connection. Their efforts spearheaded the formalization of the field of psychoneuroimmunology.

Meanwhile, a young neuroscientist named Candace Pert had made an important discovery at Johns Hopkins University in Baltimore. She found that there were receptors (combination speakers and receivers) for messages from the brain all over the surface membranes of cells in the immune system. Clearly, this meant the two systems were communicating with each other: "Why," asked Pert, "would nature have installed speakers if no one was broadcasting any music?"

She went on to do more work, with Michael Rupp, a collaborator at the National Institute of Mental Health, and confirmed that, indeed, certain white blood cells were equipped with molecular antennas tuned specifically to receive messages from the brain. Pert and Rupp saw that these messenger molecules were biochemical messengers that can affect emotions by facilitating a constant exchange of information throughout the brain and body. She also saw that these receptors to brain messages are the same ones used by viruses to enter cells. Therefore, she concluded, emotional fluctuations may determine whether the virus will be able to enter the cell and make us sick or be thwarted in the attempt.[19]

Only a decade ago, an editorial in the *New England Journal of Medicine* ridiculed the emerging work of psychoneuroimmunologists. Six years later, though, that same journal essentially reversed itself by publishing a watershed report showing direct links between stress and the common cold. Robert Ader, the researcher with the dying mice who helped galvanize the movement twenty years ago, observed that "the reaction of the scientific community has gone from 'It's impossible' to 'We knew it all along.' "[20]

Many health scientists now believe that the nervous system, the immune system, and the endocrine system are so closely linked that they form a single regulatory network in the body. The legitimacy of body-mind medicine was underscored in 1992 when the National Institutes of Health established an alternative medicine research group. That group is helping to forge stronger links between mainstream and complementary approaches to promoting health and managing illness. The NIH and an increasing number of practitioners know that germs are most likely to cause diseases when your body is too weakened, by workplace stress or by other factors, to fight them off.

It's All in the Family

The mind and body do the same dance.
—MARGARET KEMENY

Thanks to the work begun by psychoneuroimmunologists and other early practitioners of behavioral and psychosomatic medicine, it's now clear that five different body systems are affected by your reactions to what's happening to you in your career—the nervous system, the immune system, the endocrine system, the cardiovascular system, and the musculoskeletal system. What they communicate to each other determines a great deal about how well you are able to hold on to your health in the face of career crises and dilemmas.

The Nervous System

The nervous system keeps your organs in balance. Like the other systems in the body, the nervous system, consisting primarily of the brain, the spinal cord, the nerves, and the ganglia, helps the various organs to stay in relative balance with each other. "Messenger molecules" called neurotransmitters travel by way of nerve fibers or the bloodstream throughout the body. So all-inclusive is the effect of our mental states that subjects with multiple personality disorder often have within them an assortment of different ailments, which are activated according to which personality is in charge of the organism at any point in time. That is, one of the personalities may have asthma, another diabetes, and another lower back pain, and the symptoms will be manifested only when that particular personality is temporarily dominant.[21]

Cognition (what you think about things, how you interpret situations) and emotions (the feelings you're having) sit as copilots at the controls of your nervous system. Together they tell your body how to respond. When you expect something to hurt, it does; when you assume the pain will be mild, it usually is. A famous nineteenth-century demonstration of the physical effects of our assumptions was accomplished when researchers were able to trigger attacks of breathlessness in asthmatics who were allergic to roses, simply by presenting them with a paper rose.

Two contrasting psychological traits, self-efficacy and learned helplessness, seem to have a significant effect on how susceptible you'll be to illness and pain of various sorts. *Self-efficacy*, a term coined by social psychologist Albert Bandura at the University of California, is the belief that you'll be equal to the tasks you set for yourself. When you have it, not only are you more successful, but you also seem to be better able to ward off infections and other debilitating conditions. Learned helplessness, on the other hand, limits your effectiveness and predisposes you to a variety of physical and emotional problems, such as depression, recurrent infections, and a worsening of chronic conditions. When your own proclivity to learned helplessness is exacerbated by workplace stressors, your nervous system often gets other members of the "family" involved to cause you one or more physical problems.

The Immune System

Your immune system watches for invaders. Your immune system can be likened to a Patriot missile defense system, detecting incoming dangers and destroying them. The many unusual infections associated with AIDS are examples of what happens when the immune system is compromised. But the common cold, flu, and other infections are also all outcomes of weakened systems, diminished by such factors as fatigue and chronic or acute career distress.

When psychoneuroimmunologists first turned to people rather than rodents to test their theories, they focused on individuals who had endured intensely distressing events, such as astronauts at the end of a mission, survivors of a seventy-seven-hour noise and sleep deprivation event, and men and women who had recently been widowed. As expected, all of these groups evidenced depressed immune functioning as a result of what they had experienced.[22]

Numerous studies since then have shown repeatedly that the fighting power of the immune system, as measured directly by criteria such as antibodies in saliva and the activity of NK (natural killer) cells and T cells in the peripheral blood supply, and indirectly by evidence of infections, is clearly linked to your reaction to the events of your daily life. Here are just a few examples of the many interrelationships uncovered.

- People who reported a drop in self-control and confidence had a measured decrease in T cells, which attack specific microbic invaders.[23]
- Subjects who were feeling happy had stronger immune factors in their saliva than those who were unhappy.[24]
- Just before exams, students experienced attacks of trench mouth when bacteria overpowered weary infection-fighting cells.[25]
- People grieving the loss of a loved one showed reductions in immune-system fighting capability.[26]
- Harvard students judged "poor copers" in terms of dealing

with upsetting situations had many fewer NK cells than the "good copers."[27]

- Workers who believed they had no control over the pace and conditions of their jobs had higher levels of stress hormones and decreased immune effectiveness.[28]

The evidence is clear: when you're unhappy, distraught, feeling under siege, or worrying what might be happening next at work, you're very likely undercutting the fighting force of your immune system. What's also clear from the research, however, is that you have choices about how to respond to these stressors. You could give up on yourself. You could rail at your boss and others you hold responsible for what's happening at work. Or you could strategize ways to find the elusive (but surely present) opportunities in the problems you're facing. This final, preferred mode of response is much more likely to keep your immune system functioning well.

The Endocrine System

Your endocrine system is sensitive to all your thoughts and feelings. Your endocrine system also keeps you in balance and maintains your readiness to respond to internal and external stressors. The endocrine glands secrete behavior-regulating hormones directly into the bloodstream. When you are chronically stressed because of work and demands, your hormones no longer ebb and flow normally. Rather, they stay high, potentially impairing your body's ability to heal. Then the loop comes back around again, it seems, as the fact of not feeling well becomes an additional stressor, and your illness and stress hormones reinforce each other even more.

Like other branches of the family in your body, your endocrines are sensitive to everything you think and feel. What's more, they pour out immune-repressing stress hormones such as cortisol when you're depressed, angry, or feeling out of control. Studies have shown that the best way to keep your endocrine system in good working condition is by maintaining a predictable routine, which includes enough rest, exercise, affection, and feelings of control. That can be a tall order in stress-filled work settings.

The Cardiovascular System

Your cardiovascular system follows orders from your nervous system. Your cardiovascular system is quite reactive to proddings from your nervous system. Heart functions are easily affected not only by physical factors, such as exercise and diet, but also by emotions, such as fear and anger. Stressors of all kinds can elevate blood pressure and induce sudden constriction of the coronary arteries. When you are passive or angry in stressful work situations, you put incredible pressure on this hardworking delivery and maintenance system.

The good news about your cardiovascular system is that it's very receptive to body-mind interventions such as relaxation techniques, meditation, visualization, and psychotherapy. Surgical patients, for instance, who are coached to visualize blood moving away from the site of a wound or an operation are able to reduce significantly the amount of bleeding. In work settings, people are able to limit the negative cardiovascular effects of stress through a variety of techniques. When you cope effectively with stressful work situations, by managing your interpretations of events or by visualizing yourself succeeding in a demanding assignment, your heart and blood vessels keep functioning quite smoothly.

The Musculoskeletal System

Your musculoskeletal system has "first-alert" capabilities. Your musculoskeletal system of bones and muscles is also logged onto your "BodyNet" (as in "Internet"), participating constantly in the lively exchange of information about how well everyone is working together. Your muscles are actually a great "first-alert" system when you allow them to be. When you're working too hard, or keeping your negative feelings about a project at the office to yourself, or doubting yourself again, chances are they'll be trying to get you to pay attention by tensing up and causing you pain.

But your muscles are important for more than sending out warning signals. Muscle mass and strength, which you can maintain only through regular exercise, keep you feeling strong in many ways—and therefore have a lot to do with how much energy and optimism you'll be able to bring to demanding or stressful work situations. "After my morning walk, it's as if my body and I are on the same team," one busy executive commented. "That's why I schedule in a walk somehow every day, even when I'm traveling on business." When you allow the demands of your career to eat away your exercise time, you give up one of the most effective energy-builders in the world.

Listen and Learn

Emotions [are] the bridge between the mental and the physical, or the physical and the mental. It's either way.
—Candace Pert

How does all this relate to what happens at work? The connection is simple. When you're feeling anxious, angry, doubtful, or lonely because of what's happening at work, your nervous system informs all the other systems of your body. Those other systems in turn mete out a range of painful "sentences." Feeling out of control in your work, feeling like a failure, or forcing yourself to do work you don't really value or like all can diminish your likelihood of success and compromise your health.

Fighting toxicity isn't simple, because like all other complexities of modern life, the factors are both interdependent and highly variable. In general, four essential elements to consider are

- Your beliefs, temperament, and life stage
- The fit between your present needs and the demands of your job

- The lifestyle choices you're making, because of employer pressures or your own habits
- The attitudes and demands of your employer

All of these intertwine in various ways to influence how healthy you stay. It's seldom possible to isolate one cause of toxicity at work. For instance, a difficult boss pairs up with a negative-thinking employee. The employee is burned out on the job she's held for twenty years and can't stop inhaling chips and salsa and margaritas after work each night because she's so conflicted about possibly losing the job she hates. She stumbles in to work late many mornings, while the boss keeps a "paper trail" of her sloppy work habits and frequent sick days and applies more pressure. Or perhaps a quiet, slower-paced employee, who feels time is passing him by and really wants to win the lottery so he can spend his time writing novels, gets transferred into a unit with a demanding, fast-moving boss, who requires people to work sixty hours a week to keep up with her. Soon he has tension headaches and is missing work most Mondays.

As you can imagine, there are many possible combinations. Therefore, you'll need to become aware of and learn to assess the different factors for yourself, independently and cumulatively. For the rest of your working life, be that ten years or fifty, being able to diagnose your own work dissatisfactions will be a critical health-maintenance tool. Once you learn to pinpoint your own incongruities, and to take the corrective steps to which your discoveries lead you, you will be able to restore (or perhaps have for the first time) the health and happiness you deserve.

It's such a fascinating circle: Your mind affects how you experience your work, and your work in turn colors your feelings and thoughts about yourself in the world. Those reactions then instruct all the systems of your body about how to behave, individually and with each other. This is an extended family of systems that always share information with each other, whether you want them to or not. When your career feels problematic—because you've put yourself in a situation that just doesn't fit, or because the demands of your job seem impossible to meet, the delicate balance of this crucial ecosystem is disrupted. But when you decide to listen to your bodily symptoms as helpful messages telling you that it's time to *change* and *grow* in your career, quite positive things can happen.

3. Dancing with Dinosaurs and Dragons

If fate throws a knife at you, there are two ways of catching it—by the blade or by the handle. —ORIENTAL PROVERB

Sure, workplaces are toxic—the things happening there have never happened in quite this same way before. Adding to the organizational stressors of the moment, moreover, are the behaviors of some of the people there. Consider, for instance, the following scenarios:

It's Monday morning and you're a little late, as it took longer than expected to bid farewell to your visiting in-laws and fight the traffic crossing the bridge. Your head is pounding. Head down so as not to shake your brains too much, you are moving down the hall carefully toward the coffee station, when you find your boss heading in your direction. She's invisible most of the time, thankfully, but this is the morning she's chosen to be in your path, asking for that totally useless report she had requested but that you had decided to ignore. Her view of what you should be doing with your job and hers couldn't be more different. Even on a good day you can't imagine the need for the elaborate, old-fashioned paper charts she wants you to keep, when all the information she needs is on-line. It makes you furious to use your time helping her keep her distance from the computer. And this morning especially is not the time you want to be confronted with this anachronistic request.

Mort's response to employee suggestions and concerns is usually a resounding "Stop whining." You're faced with his dragonesque qualities today because you've come to ask for flexible time next week while your son is having surgery. He lets you know that your son's health is not his problem—but getting the quarterly reports out is. You offer to work longer hours this week, and you tell him that someone else in the department has volunteered to help out next week. He lets you know that all this tinkering with the schedule seems thoroughly unprofessional to him, and that if you really cared about your job, you'd have made arrangements apart from work. You leave his office torn between the desire to turn your neighbor's Doberman loose on him and the sick feeling that maybe he's right and you really aren't professional enough. On the way home, you begin a slow, obsessive recall of all the times in your life when you weren't able to quite meet the expectations of various authority figures.

Nell is your colleague, and you suspect she has never met a deadline in her life. That would be all right if she worked alone. But on your team, her tendency to put things off until the last minute and then zip in for a brilliant but tension-filled photo finish is a stressor for everyone. Nell gets herself (and everyone around her) into trouble by having more ideas than she knows what to do with. You are a responsible, organized person who finds this erratic behavior particularly hard to take—so much so that you usually come down with a nasty cold every time you and Nell are finishing up a project together.

Let's Get Physical:
The Top Thirteen Signals from Your Body

Mind and body are inextricably linked, and their second-by-second interaction exerts a profound influence upon health and illness. —KEN PELLETIER

You're not the only one who experiences your feelings in your body. We all have quite individualized menus of physical symptoms and what they mean to us. As someone who spent hours incarcerated at my grandparents' dining room table while a contest of wills ensued about whether I had to eat my green beans (a contest I always lost eventually), I know that whenever I feel nauseated, my body's telling me that I'm being pressured into doing something I don't really want to do. My nausea has been very helpful to me in understanding my own tendency to procrastinate. Once I had figured out that I sometimes felt sick when a project had been hanging around calling my name for a while, I realized that I procrastinate most about the things I didn't want to take on in the first place. So I have learned to wait a period of time before taking on or dreaming up new assignments (when there's a choice, that is) and to say yes far less frequently. I've felt less nauseated and have fewer projects in the Overwhelming Guilt Pile as a result. You of course have your own list of physical signals. Here are some symptoms that people frequently talk about in my office. Check off any that seem familiar to you:

_____ Fatigue that doesn't go away with a couple good nights' sleep

_____ Insomnia

_____ Dizziness/light-headedness

_____ Headaches

_____ Nausea

_____ Allergies/breathing difficulties

_____ Skin problems

_____ Recurrent colds/flu/infections

_____ Muscle aches/stiffness

_____ Digestive-tract problems

_____ Back pain

_____ Increased menstrual difficulties

_____ Swollen glands/sore throat

Your body is probably only doing its job—letting you know that something isn't quite right, and telling you to figure it out somehow. Don't ignore the message: get busy identifying what needs fixing before it makes you any sicker.

People Can Be Toxic, Too

EVIL. That which one believes of others. It is a sin to believe
evil of others, but it is seldom a mistake.   —H. L. MENCKEN

In the workplaces where most of you report every day, there are
any number of people who make it difficult to do what you need to
do. Difficult people show up at all levels—there are very likely
bosses, peers, and subordinates causing you trouble. Figuring out
how to handle these people from a position of reason and control,
rather than desperation, can go a long way toward keeping down the
levels of toxicity in your day.

Take the case of Brian, whose catalog idea was stolen by his colleague Lydia. Brian had just arrived at a meeting to discuss the new
promotion campaign for the fall catalog, wondering how the various
functions would be handled. Who would be the team leader for this
one? he asked himself. And how would the strategy be decided?
The meeting had barely begun when Lydia, the new person on the
team, grabbed the floor and launched into a detailed discussion of
the idea Brian had mentioned to her in passing last week, claiming
it as her own and proposing that she be the person to lead the team
this time, "just to get some practice and catch up with everyone
else." She then proceeded to hand out color charts and graphs of
Brian's idea. The boss fell for it, and asked Lydia to head up the
team. Brian, blindsided, sat there, fuming. Pretty soon he left the
meeting and went to take three ibuprofens for his raging headache.
Luckily, his desk drawer was well-stocked.

Once Brian had ruled out homicide as the treatment of choice,
he considered a range of options for dealing with this situation. The
first thing Brian had to do was acknowledge that hurtful, unfair,
toxic events and situations do occur with regularity. People do take
credit for others' work and steal others' accounts, clients, and ideas.
They also sabotage others, discriminate against people who are different from them, hurt others' feelings, discount others' achievements, and cause fights unnecessarily. It's also likely that someone
on your team or in your office consistently doesn't deliver, and

nothing happens to correct the situation. Or perhaps you're too far down in the hierarchy to have your ideas heard or get credit as you'd like. And of course egos are miles wide and high. Lots of workplaces seem unsafe or out of control because of these and other kinds of behaviors and situations. Brian wasn't alone. But his next step was to calm himself down, so that he could plan his moves strategically.

Bosses cause problems in lots of ways also. Sometimes you feel your boss is less qualified than you are, and sometimes it's true. Some bosses are control freaks, while others are too unclear about what they want and need from you. Some have trouble with boundaries and are alternately too close and too demanding. Other bosses are threatened by their best performers, while some are stuck in yesterday and don't know it.

Much of the dragonesque behavior in toxic workplaces has accelerated with more stressful economic conditions. Nobody's exactly cheerful about giving up their security, losing a job, or doing three jobs for one job's pay. Mike, whose supervisory units tripled when the two other line supervisor positions were eliminated, put it this way: " 'Re-engineering,' what a crock term that is. Why don't they just call it 'demolition derby'?" He feels caught in the catch-22 of needing his job and yet finding it impossible to do. The workers on his lines find him alternately dejected and rageful. He's hard to be around, and even a little scary sometimes. Mike is not the only angry "survivor" out there making life hard for the people around him.

Some people at work are dinosaurs, some are dragons, and some are both. Whatever the style, however, the only way to keep the toxicity quotient low for you is to accept these hassles as part of the business of working with people in a difficult situation, and view them as challenges rather than as assaults. If you persist in letting them feel like warfare, battle wounds are inevitable. If you choose to view them as strategic challenges (after a little rolling of the eyes and silently hurling a few of your favorite epithets for relief, that is), then you will have passed another round of qualifying tests for the great game of surviving toxicity. The next lesson, then, is deducing whether the assaults happening to you have anything to do with your own buttons and hot spots.

Keep in mind the interactive nature of workplace stress. Dinosaurs and dragons couldn't hook you if you didn't take your own proclivities to work. If you don't believe me, ask everybody in your office to watch the same provocative film one weekend, and then gather on Monday morning to talk about it. Ask everybody what they thought the film was about, who were the good guys and bad guys, whether it ended correctly, what parts they found hard to watch, and so on. You'll probably be wondering if you all saw the same film by the end of the discussion. And that's just the point—we're *not* seeing the same film every day at work, even though we're working in the same office.

What's Pushing Your Buttons?

We have met the enemy and he is us.   —WALT KELLY

We seem to drag a long bag of old laundry from earlier experiences wherever we go as adults. There is a therapist's adage: "Whenever two people make love, six people climb into bed together," and that was written long before divorced and reconfigured families greatly increased the numbers of parent figures on each side. The same formula applies to work. Given the numbers and different types of parents, grandparents, siblings, teachers, counselors, coaches, clerics, and employers most of us dealt with in the harrowing process of learning to produce and achieve, most of us sit at work each day with at least twenty people crowding us in our chair and sprawling over the desk. Our interactions with these folks over the years have often left us with lots of "hot spots," which get activated by toxic work situations. These hot spots manifest themselves in the nearly constant internal chatter that follows us throughout the day. We bring into adulthood a range of sensitivities to issues such as authority, criticism, competition, space, and self-worth. Here are some of the messages people find playing on their internal tape decks when they force themselves to stop to listen. Notice the ones that resonate for you:

- "It's not fair."
- "I'm not getting my share again."
- "I always get left."
- "Nobody listens to me."
- "They're picking on me."
- "Something always gets messed up."
- "You can't count on anyone."
- "It's never quite good enough."
- "I don't really fit in here."
- "Just come out swinging."
- "I always make a fool of myself."
- "Nobody cares what I think."
- "Nobody understands."
- "You're crowding me."
- "It's got to be perfect."
- "People are just so stupid."
- "Don't boss me around."

Our friend Brian, for instance, turned up the volume and found "It's not fair" and "They're picking on me" tapes blasting away. Lydia's sneaky behavior was not acceptable by any standard. But Brian's difficulty with letting go of his hurt and outrage so he could figure out a productive response came mostly from his interpretation of that betrayal as a recapitulation of old family patterns when, as the "different one" in his family and the smallest kid in his class, he had repeatedly been beaten out by others. For Brian, a major part of not getting stuck there yet again was seeing it for what it was and deciding to edit that script through a referral for brief cognitive therapy. When he finally went to Lydia to make it clear that she had better not try any such end runs again, he spoke from a place of strength, rather than little-boy frustration. That's the good news about problematic cognitions—they can be changed!

So try "squinting" back into your own earlier family, school, and employment experiences. That means imagining yourself as you were at an earlier time, peering intently into buried memories about yourself. What problems turned up for you again and again in your family or in school? What debilitating messages were playing for you then? They're probably still alive and well. The trick is that they're hard to see or hear by yourself. When it seems that other people in the group aren't responding the same way you are to a person or situation, it should be a clue that one of your individual hot spots has snagged you. You'll probably need to talk to someone else who knows you well—a friend, family member, colleague, or counselor—to help you understand how your own hot spots might be getting in your way now. They're nothing to be ashamed about—we all have them. But when your hot spots get activated, you are sucked into the "irrational zone" and it's harder to marshal the strategic planfulness you need to implement sound, centered solutions.

And What If You Are Sometimes a Dragon?

We can't be more sensitive to pleasure without being more sensitive to pain.   —ALAN WATTS

It's been said that the people who are the most likely to be controlling and critical are middle managers, for they're the ones who will be displaced or lose power if workers get more influence in organizations. I think there's some truth in that structural analysis, but I also believe that there are psychological variables in operation. Dragons do pop up at all levels in organizations.

The theories of Swiss psychoanalyst Alice Miller are very revealing. Throughout the prodigious body of Miller's works, the theme of the long-lasting and often pernicious effects of childhood experience plays out in various ways.

Miller explains with great insight the compulsion to be controlling. Every one of us has experienced some degree of disappointment, unkindness, neglect, or pain as a child. In our adult lives, says Miller, we have one of two choices about what we do with this pain, which is of course quite "alive" in the recesses of our unconscious mind. We can pull it up into our conscious awareness, through such vehicles as psychotherapy, dream analysis, intense conversations, sharing slivers of our memories with loved ones, or making art. Once exposed to the healing light of conscious discussion or artful display, painful memories can be understood in context and the pain can be excised to some degree. But it is often an upsetting process, and people do not suffer psychological upset easily. Too many people, particularly those drawn to positions of power, keep themselves from knowing about the pain they endured as children by unconsciously identifying with the oppressor. This identification compels them to adhere to strict, rigid standards, at work and in their personal lives.[1]

Once I had read Miller, and was jolted with the truth of it, I began to observe more and more people who seemed to be reenacting their own unresolved (and unacknowledged) childhood pain. I went to meetings with managers who practically pounded the table insisting that workers were getting away with too much and needed to be monitored at all times. I listened to faculty members in various schools and colleges who seemed obsessed with the need for ever more rigor to put their students to the test. They were, of course, convinced that students were getting less and less capable all the time, and needing somebody to be tougher on them—even at Ivy League institutions.

I talked with doctors who were enraged that residents and medical students training under them dared to want more balanced lives, when they had been forced to endure so much more during their own internships and residencies. And I talked to hundreds of workers, most of them experiencing some kind of emotional or physical distress, who could trace the problems in their work units to a seeming compulsion on the part of their supervisors to keep them in a regulated, submissive state.

These compulsions are usually obvious to observers, but seldom perceptible to the people caught in their grip. Since the purpose of a psychological "defense" is to keep early experience and pain safely under wraps, how would you know if you, your partner, or your boss were afflicted with this syndrome of excessive control? The following questions have helped others to alert themselves to the possibility that some painful old memories might be needing to break out, in order to allow them to be more open to change and collaboration. Pose these questions to yourself or someone you know—and then find someone you can trust to talk with about them.

SUPERCONTROLLER SURVEY

For each of the following questions, circle the number that seems to apply best (1 = very little, 2 = somewhat, 3 = quite a bit, 4 = a very great deal). When you've responded to all ten statements, add the scores to get a total.

- How much does it bother you when people seem to get away with not doing a job right? 1 2 3 4
- How much would you do to force co-workers or subordinates to maintain the highest standards at all times? 1 2 3 4
- How much do you long for the way things used to be and get irritated at the new freedoms you see around you? 1 2 3 4
- How much do you either tune out or get angry when people complain about what's wrong? 1 2 3 4
- How much does disorder of any sort bother you? 1 2 3 4
- How much do you think it's the case that people talk about their feelings to avoid taking on adult responsibilities? 1 2 3 4
- How much do you find yourself getting angry or impatient easily? 1 2 3 4
- How much do people tell you that you're too much of a perfectionist? 1 2 3 4
- How much do you want things done your way? 1 2 3 4
- How much do you think it's right for people to learn lessons the hard way? 1 2 3 4

If you get a score of twenty-five or more on these ten questions, you're probably a good candidate for causing workplace stress, for yourself and for others. You'll cause it for yourself by turning your high standards and unforgiving style on your own performance. If you're managing others, you'll cause it by contributing to a demanding, hostile, and perfectionistic atmosphere.

This is not to say that quality and high standards are not important. What matters is how angry and inflexible you are about getting there. Hostility and rigidity are particularly problematic because they seldom deliver the desired result over the long term. Research shows again and again that the leaders who get the most from their troops are those who have high standards, but also coach, support, and affirm them along the way. Supercontroller bosses, therefore, often find that they've inadvertently caused the lackluster outcome they most wanted to avoid.

Are there solutions to be tried if you've found yourself in the "potential oppressor" category? Of course there are—the point to being alive is to keep on growing. Just talking will help at first, along with all the other strategies for self-awareness and change in this book. You might also want to consider an appointment with a counselor to put your responses in perspective. And what can you do if you work for or with a supercontroller who's causing you grief or pain? For supercontrollers, and for their colleagues and subordinates, here are some strategies to help you cope.

The Choice Is Yours

Is the system going to flatten you out and deny your humanity, or are you going to be able to make use of the system to the attainment of human purposes?   —Joseph Campbell

When you're hearing the music start up for what you fear will be another toxic waltz, day after day, it's hard to remember that you have choices about how to respond—but that's the key to taking care of yourself. You can apply a simple three-step process:

- *Check out your hot spots:* What old stuff of yours is being exacerbated by the events of the day? Are you willing to own your half of the dance and resist getting thrown into crisis mode?
- *Monitor your own self-defeating behaviors:* Do you feel tempted to do anything irrational, like screaming at your boss, firing someone without documentation, deleting a week's worth of work from the computer in a state of rage, or collapsing into a depressed state? If the answer is yes, *don't.* Consider calling someone to help you regain your sense of equilibrium.
- *Select a strategy:* From the eight strategies described below, pick several that you think could be helpful now. If the first one or two you choose don't work, keep trying until one of them does.

Strategies for Preserving Choice

1. Control the intensity. Sometimes it's clear that things aren't going to get better. For instance, a co-worker may be incurably immature or your supervisor is clearly intolerant of something about you that you can't change, such as your ethnicity, your gender, or your sexual orientation. But you want to stay in the organization, so it's up to you to manage your own perceptions and reactions. You can often manage the intensity of your responses by controlling how information reaches you. Psychological "technologies" allow you to blunt the impact of stimuli in two ways: by reducing the intensity of the stressor or by substituting positive experiences. When someone is in your face saying things that hurt, and confronting him or her right then and there doesn't seem appropriate, you can work with your imagination to put some distance between you and the stressor: you could "dim the lights," "turn down the volume," or "make the picture smaller." If your boss throws a nasty barb your way after a sales presentation, rather than constructively pointing out the strengths and weaknesses of your approach, you can imagine him talking to you from the far end of the parking lot, or from behind a closed toilet stall so you can't see his face. Do whatever it takes to escape the intensity of the moment and buy yourself some time to get into a more measured, reasonable mode.

Or you can take away the sting of an unsettling situation by overlaying it with positive associations. I knew someone, for instance, who was deathly afraid of car washes. Something about going through them, trapped in her car with brushes and belts slapping noisily amidst gushing water, pushed her panic buttons. Yet she needed a clean car to make sales calls in, and she didn't have the time or facilities to do it by hand. So she learned to park outside the car wash for a few minutes, close her eyes and breathe deeply, imagining herself on a dock at the ocean as a brisk but benign wind came up. She smelled the salt, and imagined the dock rocking gently to and fro. Once she felt submerged in those pleasant—and safe—images, she was ready to go through the car wash, experiencing it as an extension of her beachfront fantasy.

You can prepare for tough situations at work the same way. When you're heading into a difficult meeting, take a few minutes without interruptions at your desk beforehand. Imagine a place that you love, where you feel relaxed and joyful. Then picture your potential adversaries walking toward you amiably *in that environment*. In your visualization, greet them warmly, experience them as friendly and nonthreatening, and tell them you're looking forward to seeing them at the meeting. Then, as you walk into the *real* meeting, call up the visualized, positive interaction. Especially remember the calm and relaxed feelings you had. You'll be surprised how differently you'll experience the meeting.

2. Go around, not through. Another important strategy in intractable situations is to map your travel *around* rather than *through* stormy scenes. For example, if you suspect that another unit head in your organization is probably out to embarrass you at the next meeting because he disagrees with your approach to the project you're about to launch, decide whether you want to slug it out with him in public. If the answer is no, choose one of the several good reasons you have for being needed elsewhere, send your regrets and your own ideas to the project leader in writing in advance of the meeting, and avoid the confrontation. Being overly *obedient* (i.e., always doing what's expected) rather than *strategic* (having a greater impact in a different way) often gets people in the toxic soup in organizations.

3. Remember what your body needs. Another critical strategy is self-care. When things are increasingly toxic, you really need to pay attention to what your body and spirit are needing, even though that's the first thing most people forget about in hard times and has all the logic of leaving the life preservers at home because there's a storm brewing. Here are some life preservers to get you through this storm:

- Deep-breathing exercises and meditation—If you meditate in the morning and evening and use deep breathing to get centered when a dragon pokes its head into your workday, you'll be surprised at how unruffled you can stay.
- Exercise—Use some kind of physical movement or exercise to change the energy of dark moments—walking or stretching are free and easily accessible. It's simple if you keep good walking shoes in the closet at the office.
- Play—I have a Ping-Pong table in my basement to call up my endorphins (opiate-like substances in the brain that produce feelings of well-being), and I know other people who regularly find renewal in golf, some quick hands of bridge, or Scrabble.
- Laughter—This wonderfully recuperative sport of "internal jogging" is handled in Chapters 6 and 7.
- A nap or a long morning in bed—Most physicians will tell you that fatigue is the factor most likely to wear down both your physiological and psychological defenses.
- Art and music—Apollo is both the god of music and the god of medicine. There's something very therapeutic about these kinds of sensory stimulation.

4. Negotiate, don't alienate. Another helpful strategy is to bring a negotiator's mind set to situations. See negative responses, disagreements, or demands as *opportunities for negotiation.* For instance, when Connie came back from a six-month maternity leave, she was greeted by the vice president in her division telling her that he wanted her to take over leadership of a new-product development project. He told her it was because she had the expertise required, but she also knew that no one else wanted the assignment because it was risky. In her heavily male environment, all eyes were on her to see if she could still compete after becoming a mother. Taking on a visible, time-consuming project in a semi-exhausted state was about the last thing Connie wanted to do, but her political instincts told her she couldn't turn down the assignment without permanently damaging her reputation. So she decided to pair taking on the task with getting two things she wanted—more flexibility in terms of time and a good bonus if the project was successful. The VP thought the requests were fair, and it was a win-win. Connie got to work from home via fax and modem two days a week, often scheduling conference calls with people in the field and on the team in corporate headquarters, and she also got the hefty bonus she wanted when the project was a great success. It's a funny thing about win-lose situations—there never is a long-term winner. But when you use your negotiation skills to push for both you and the other side to win, the results are usually much more positive.

5. Clarify. Clarity is another simple but often-neglected strategy in the midst of toxicity. Insist that goals, expectations, and boundaries be clear and adhered to. Put things in writing whenever possible, either directly or via strategic copying to certain people on your letters and memos. Having agendas before meetings and action notes afterwards, and circulating written progress notes on important projects all have a calming, settling effect, particularly for people whose anxieties skyrocket in the face of ambiguity. It may seem that writing things down creates more work when you already have too much, but you can delegate or rotate the task. Do it wisely—ask for pithy action notes rather than formal minutes, for instance—and you'll find that the minimal effort pays off. Writing down what's been decided is also a deterrent to bosses or colleagues with a penchant to change plans mid-project—knowing that everybody has in writing what the agreements were. Clients of mine who worked for or were themselves scattershot managers have appreciated the grounding results of having to follow through on plans because they had been committed to paper. In our current workplaces, ambiguity is everywhere—whatever tiny antidotes we can provide for ourselves and others go a long way toward reducing toxins.

6. Guard against give-aways. You must also stop giving at the office again and again, particularly when you're being stalked by dinosaurs and dragons. It's shocking how many people seem to be *offering* to give it all away, which somehow has the effect of worsening the effects of the toxicity around them. The give-away artists I encounter are giving away all of the following:

- *Their time:* by not protecting their calendars; by agreeing to do tasks that won't get much in the way of results; by being the ready ear to everyone in distress and using up all their reserves in the process; by letting relationships atrophy in deference to work demands
- *Their money:* by anesthetic spending; by paying for things when they don't need to; by being afraid to ask for what's due them; by not calculating the real dollar-per-hour return on their investment of time
- *Their power:* by choosing to please rather than confront; by pretending that abuses are not happening; by sitting on their own good ideas for fear of displeasing unpredictable colleagues and supervisors; by fearing disapproval
- *Their right to their own opinions:* by being too obedient; by not saying what they know to be true; by pretending not to notice a variety of inefficiencies and bad managerial moves
- *Their peace of mind:* by doing what's expected rather than what they view as appropriate; by being a "company person" rather than relying on their own assessments of what's going on; by worrying about the organization as a whole rather than

leaving it to the people in charge (this latter act is what adult children of alcoholics do—they fret incessantly about problems that they have no power to fix)

- *Their life balance:* by staying too late and taking on extra projects to satisfy an insatiable person or system; by valuing company opinions more than opinions at home; by forgetting what really matters.

If the way you're doing your job and responding to the toxicity at work is causing one or more of these give-away situations in your life, it's time to make some changes. Both your health and your career are on the line here.

7. Don't forget the support. Strategic support is essential too. Under stress, many people try to go solo, when what they need is others' help to see things clearly, anticipate problems, and implement good plans. It's easy to cave in as the toxins swirl around you in the swamp, and just work through the night to get an important overdue project done, for instance. That's always a bad choice: many more organizational errors get made in solo mode than in a group of smart, like-minded, supportive people. You'd be much better off to negotiate one last extension and ask one or two people you trust to help you shape the final product or make a pressing decision. Pride is often the villain here. Who among us wants to admit to feeling overwhelmed or stumped? But it's better to share your distress (selectively, of course) and get back on track midway through the project, rather than suffer through to the end with impaired judgment by yourself, make a bigger mess, and ensure that the toxins will multiply.

8. Take three daily doses of pleasure. I generally ask people who are struggling with toxicity at work to plan *three pleasures* very strategically into each day. Resistance to this unfamiliar tactic can come up in insidious ways, I've found. You tell yourself that taking time to think about pleasure when there's such important work to be done would be procrastinating or unprofessional. It seems *silly,* and so you put it off. But it's not silly at all—it's about claiming some measure of control for yourself. A pleasure doesn't have to be big and it doesn't matter what it is—it only matters that each and every day must contain *by design* three things that will pleasure you. Because *pleasure planning* is so foreign to our way of thinking about workdays, I usually have to help people prime the pump by showing them a list of possibilities. See if anything on the list below gets any ideas going for you:

_____ Walking at lunch time

_____ Sending jokes or funny stories via e-mail to colleagues

_____ Setting aside time to ponder a project that really interests you

_____ Going window-shopping at lunch or after work

_____ Reading the article that's been calling out to you

_____ Going to a meeting where people you enjoy will be present

_____ Stopping by to exchange jokes or stories with someone

_____ Taking home a video or a new CD

_____ Calling someone special you haven't contacted in a while

_____ Calling someone for a spontaneous lunch date

_____ Taking a bunch of flowers to your office

_____ Dressing up so you feel special that day

_____ Taking a tape or CD player to work and treating yourself to some favorite music during the day

_____ Working out in the gym or jogging before or after work

_____ Meeting a colleague from another organization for a relaxing sharing of information and ideas

_____ Trying a new or old favorite restaurant for lunch—take time to savor the tastes and/or ambience you like

_____ Playing humorous tapes or an audio tape of the book you've been wanting to read on the way to work

_____ Inviting your whole team out to lunch

_____ Taking a meditation or a creative-visualization break

_____ Taking a crossword puzzle break

_____ Posting funny sayings or cartoons on your office door and seeing how people respond

_____ Playing with toys you keep in the office—Slinkys, Play-Doh, a basketball hoop on your trash basket

_____ Meeting someone at a favorite coffee bar

_____ Buying a new pen (or gratifying whatever your own particular fetish is)

_____ Playing a game or two on the computer between tasks

_____ Watching the fish in your aquarium for a while, especially during a stressful phone call (surgical patients heal better after surgery when they've stared at fish for a while—it helps with handling difficult situations, too)

After a while these pleasurable moments will happen without your planning it, but at the start you'll need to structure in these things. It's amazing how hard it is to get many people to commit to taking care of themselves and staying energized, even when research shows that "feeling more alive" will enhance job performance. It often seems they'd rather be disappointed and used up and then get to moan about it. This can get you sympathy and connection the first few times, but people soon distance from perpetually negative colleagues or friends, leaving you lonelier and less effective than before.

Symptoms, Hot Spots, Strategies: Keeping Toxicity at Bay

It always comes back to the same necessity. Go deep enough and there is a bedrock of truth, however hard.
—May Sarton

So it's as simple as this:

• Look out for signals that come as symptoms. Welcome them, don't bludgeon or ignore them.

- Spend some time discovering your own hot spots; commit to controlling (rather than being controlled by) them. Expect that the greater the toxicity of the situation, the more likely you are to experience flash points.
- Choose and invent strategies—there is no such thing as an impossible problem. If the eight strategies I've suggested don't work for you, develop your own. If you can't change the toxic situation, you can certainly change how you are choosing to manage it.

Unfortunately, some people are drawn to workplace toxicity like moths to the flame. Given their family histories, turmoil feels comfortable. Stubbornly, they just keep on inviting crises and insults, unconsciously refusing to get out, when they could with some good strategizing and determination. *Victim* seems to be their favorite role. If you think you might fall into that category, don't give up on this strategy list until you've found some relief or have devised some positive substitutes of your own. To ensure that you won't give up, ask a friend or colleague to take the journey with you, and you can keep tabs on each other. *Martyr* is another favorite role when the dragons are roaming around. The martyrs do the impossible tasks without complaining and never think to mention the fact that the emperor/dragon might be naked. Martyrdom is seductive: you get to appear to be the "good guy," doing what's asked and never demanding anything for yourself. But *martyrs* and *victims* have the same effect at work. They grease the skids for dysfunctional organizations to keep rolling along, perpetuating dishonesty and never confronting the behaviors and attitudes that keep real colleagueship, trust, and team-building from happening. And the real end result? Employees get sick, and organizations falter in the marketplace—hardly what anyone intended.

Even if we were to implement every organizational detoxifier in every management book or journal on the shelf, there would still be individual dinosaurs and dragons getting in the way of your work. So now is the time to get over wishing that that were not the case. You probably didn't get "placed" in the model family, and there isn't any such thing as a model employer either. Even the mythic good guys you read about have warts.

Here's the only thing you can count on—your ability to keep toxicity in perspective, and manage it when it gets in your way. This is not to say that you should just suffer and "make the most of it" if you're in a situation that really doesn't work for you. Changing jobs is an option that is tougher to do these days, but possible. Of course, you must remember that if you leave without understanding your own hot spots, they just get stuffed back into that bag and move to your new job with you. Once the novelty wears off, they'll be heating up more regularly. In a new job or the same job, managing toxic situations and toxic people is never easy. But it's always possible. Keep reading in this book, and if anything you're reading makes you a little uncomfortable, that's a sure sign that you need to read it again.

PART II

MAKING MAJOR CHANGES: DESIGNING A NONTOXIC LIFE

4. How About a Prison Break?

Be not afraid of growing slowly, be afraid only of standing still. —CHINESE PROVERB

"I just feel so stuck." That's probably the lament I hear more than any other. Many times people mean that their employer has them stuck; there is simply "no place to go" in the organization. Other times, they mean that they have financial obligations and responsibilities keeping them from cutting loose and doing what they'd really like to do. More often than not, however, I see people stuck because they keep getting in their own way.

Stepping off the Path of Least Resistance

The leap into new places is never made in comfort.
—MARVIN WEISBORD

Those of us who live in the country know what happens to steep gravel driveways in wet weather. Once the surface gets a groove in it, by a plow in a snowstorm or a truck coming up on a rainy day, that groove wears deeper and deeper. Each time it rains, the channel becomes a little wider and deeper. Pretty soon, the water, which follows the path of least resistance, has its own plan for your driveway.

That *path of least resistance* may be at work in your career as well. The choices you make every day begin to wear grooves which become harder and harder to escape. Some ruts are deeper than others, but all of them can do damage to your career. Let's look at two: a generalized *negativity*, and something I call *Recurrent Career Adversity Syndrome* (RCAS).

Negativity: The Same Old Sour Story?

People at high risk for heart attack go through life striving without joy, in the manner of Sisyphus, the character from Greek mythology who was condemned to push a heavy stone to the top of a hill only to have it always roll back down. —Stewart Wolf

Negativity is obviously the absence of optimism, what psychologists call negative cognitive appraisal—the art of continually telling yourself that success is impossible, that you'll fight to the finish line and then lose. It's very easy to fall into, or at least it was for Madeline, a perennially unemployed physical therapist. Once an excellent student, Madeline had finished near the top of her physical therapy class, and had even published a paper with one of her professors just after graduation. She was hired at a very prestigious hospital, and seemed to be on her way to a great career. But she hit some rocks early on when she got sick and felt that her supervisors wanted her to come back to work too soon. That's when her negativity seemed to just take over. From that point on, she began changing jobs, moving from one clinic to another, searching for a place that would be more understanding and less demanding. She was relieved, finally, to be able to take ten years off for parenting. But then the kids were in school, and Madeline's husband was pushing her to go to work again. Madeline came to me several times a year between her fortieth and forty-fifth birthdays, each time complaining that things were worse than ever. She had recurrent back problems, an aging mother who required constant care, and two sons who were regularly in trouble with authorities. Each time

Madeline had gotten close to landing a job, some new physical problem or family emergency had forced her to miss a deadline or cancel an interview and knock herself out of the running.

"It's always been like this," she said one day. "I guess I'm just not supposed to find work I like." Madeline's story is not one with a happy ending as of this writing: at the last session we had, Madeline left me with a comment that has come to epitomize for me the worst of how negative thinking limits people's lives. She said, "Soon my mother will be gone and it will be my turn to be taken care of; then all this bad luck with my career will seem irrelevant."

Sometimes being sick or sickly is the result of finding some indirect power in being unequal to certain tasks (like finding or keeping a job). Madeline was the daughter of a physician who had been away from home most of the time when she was a child. The one thing Madeline knew would get his attention was for her to be sick. It was also effective with her mother, whose attention was riveted on issues of illness. It's as if Madeline's mother caught a case of "Medical Student Syndrome" from her husband when he was in medical school—interpreting whatever she was feeling as the symptoms of the illness being studied—and had never quite recovered from an ongoing tendency to somatize.

For Madeline, then, there was control in being sick. She got attention, she held a powerful veto over activities and events, and she didn't have to take risks. This syndrome is not limited to medical families. I see many people using real or potential illness as a way to organize their fears.

"I can't be expected to concentrate on finding work I'd really like," they tell themselves. "I have to be careful of my health, you know." And so they have an excuse not to take responsibility for things that might be difficult, such as going for a promotion, making plans for more education, starting a new venture, or leaving a spent relationship. Those who concentrate almost exclusively on documenting and managing physical symptoms often seem able to absolve themselves of the requirement to be in charge of their own lives.[1]

While Madeline is perhaps the most severely stuck person I've worked with, her situation is not unusual. Negative thinking pervades the workplace. It feeds on itself, saps energy, and causes people to feel stuck in situations that could be potentially rewarding. There's the department head biding time until retirement, criticizing everyone's work. There's the cost-cutting COO known throughout the organization as "the Slasher." And there's the clerk in shipping who is convinced that management is just waiting a little longer to replace them all with robots.

Social psychologist Martin Seligman is one of the world's leading experts on negative thinking and optimism. His book, *Learned Optimism*, is a must for really negative thinkers or the people who live with them. He observes that

> habitual pessimistic thoughts . . . not only grab our attention; they circle unceasingly through our minds. By their very nature they will not allow themselves to be forgotten. They are primitive, biological reminders of needs and of dangers. . . . But in modern life, these primitive reminders can get in our way, subverting our performance and spoiling the quality of our emotional life.[2]

Negative thinking starts early. As children, we tell ourselves stories to make sense of life's events. Those stories—positive or negative—can last a lifetime. According to Seligman, we choose among three pairs of qualities to explain situations that happen to us:

- Is this a permanent or temporary problem?
- Is this a universal or specific situation?
- Did I cause this or did someone do it to me?

Suppose, for instance, you've been passed over for a much-desired promotion. Understandably, you feel disappointed, angry, frustrated, sad. You then have the different explanatory "scripts" available to you.

Negative thinkers are likely to conclude the following: "Being rejected for that promotion is a permanently hopeless problem. It means that I'll never have a shot at management, because I'm just not good enough. It must be due to some flaw in me—hence things are out of my control." Optimists, on the other hand, are more likely to see it this way: "This is a specific problem caused by a temporary miscommunication with my manager. I can, however, work it out before the next promotion opportunity comes along." Now, which explanation do you think seems more likely to galvanize someone to purposeful and effective action?

Of course, there is always the possibility that being passed over for promotion is a signal that you've stayed too long and it's time to move on. If that's the case, you'll still need a good supply of optimism to help you get out and on your way. If you recognize yourself as someone who has been giving away your power through negative thinking, you can use some of the suggestions scattered throughout the book in response to other problems. A basic turnaround strategy to consider is this:

1. Watch for things that make you uncomfortable—in this book, on a TV show, or in something that's said to you. Talk to yourself a bit, searching for more information about what's bringing up feelings of inadequacy, fear, or resentment for you.

2. Ask someone you trust for some gentle feedback—how does your negativity usually show itself? In what situations? Resist the urge to proclaim, "That's not true." Be grateful that your "informer" cares enough about you to be taking the risk of telling you the truth. Listen carefully.

3. Once you've got a handle on when, where, and how your negative thinking is operating, then you're ready to take it on.

Seligman suggests that you can begin the task of silencing your negative internal chatter in both immediate and longer-term ways. The short-term approach, *distraction*, is simple. When one of those thoughts sneaks in, do whatever it takes to block it. Yell "Stop!" to yourself, stamp your foot, pinch yourself, wager with your brain and agree to worry about it later. If you have a pen and paper handy, writing down your negative thoughts as you send them on their way helps to keep them away longer. The doubter's diary exercise from Chapter 3 might be helpful too.

Eventually, however, you'll want to use a longer-lasting antidote, a technique Seligman calls *disputation*. The disputation process has five parts:[3]

- Adversity
- Belief
- Consequences
- Disputation
- Energization

Let's demonstrate. You're working for a dragon of a boss who reminds you of the fifth-grade teacher you hated. Both combined perfectionism, impatience, and a critical snarl that pushes all your buttons about not being smart enough to really succeed. It's Monday and you were away for the weekend. You took the report you knew was due with you to edit, but you were having such a much-needed good time that you let it rest in your briefcase in the trunk of your car all weekend. But suddenly he's at your door, asking for the report. "What's wrong with you?" he shouts when you say you need a few more hours to wrap it up. "When will I ever get some competent help?" *Adversity* just came knocking.

Next the negative *belief*: "He's right, you know," you tell yourself. "If I were really competent, I'd have finished this last week. I know Ted would have gotten the work done on time. He's probably planning to fire me, and I wouldn't blame him. I've been a failure since the fifth grade, and I deserve to be let go."

The *consequences*: You feel nauseated again and your head is pounding. You pull the hundred-capsule bottle of ibuprofen out of your drawer and are shocked to find it almost empty. You chuck down three of them, and then put your head down on your desk.

So is that the end of it? Will you spend the rest of the day feeling lousy? Fortunately, no. Here comes *disputation*: You pick your head up off the desk and say, "Stop it." Then you continue: "Of course it would have been better to have the report ready. But he forgets that he had me on the Wilkins project all week. I put in more than forty hours on that project, because he said it was important. In the future, I'll have to ask him to prioritize projects. It's not that I'm unable to do the work; there's just too much of it. What's more, he's not going to fire me—raging around is just his style. I'm not going to let him make me sick every time he throws a tantrum."

You let yourself feel the truth and the balance of that disputation. Then comes *energization*: You feel relieved that your nausea and your headache have both subsided. You write down how you're feeling now. "I'm glad I was able to stop that negativity. Now I can get on with finishing the report. When I hand it in later this afternoon, I'll ask him about prioritizing projects so that I know where to put my energies. As for his outbursts, the only thing I can do is not let them get to me."

Try the ABCDE disputation yourself the next time a toxic situation kicks you into negative mode. Then tell some other negative thinkers about it—you could make a game of it.

Seligman and other researchers and practitioners insist that you can have control over how you explain and interpret life events. If the problem is temporary, there's very likely a light at the end of the tunnel. If it's specific, then you can probably find a solution and get on your way. And if it's external, rather than a result of your internal flaws, then you can probably strategize some solution that doesn't require a total personality overhaul. How you explain situations to yourself, therefore, determines how likely you are to feel done in by them.

Your way of seeing the world will probably stay the same unless you mount a conscious effort to exchange your negative lens for a more positive one. When Seligman and a young colleague, Melanie Burns, issued a call through a senior citizens publication for people who had kept a diary throughout adolescence and adulthood, they got access to thirty diaries. The analyses of these records of events and feelings kept intact for up to fifty years were astounding. Those people who had attributed their lack of social life as teenagers to being "unlovable," for instance, wrote as grandparents that their children and grandchildren didn't come to visit for the same reasons.[4] Their proclivity to explain life as negative and disappointing had held steady over a lifetime.

So what does that have to do with being stuck in career negativity? Everything. *Expectation edits reality.* When your job doesn't fit and you view the problem as permanent, pervasive, and personalized, it's almost impossible to find the energy to do the work of arranging a change. And so you stay stuck, spinning your wheels, and getting angry or depressed. What happens to your body then is that feelings of helplessness and hopelessness soon translate into depressed immune function. Meanwhile, the repressed rage that often accompanies feeling out of control increases cholesterol buildup and creates muscle tension that brings headaches and other kinds of pain.

Psychologist Susan Jeffers demonstrates in her workshops with women that feeling negative erodes not only your intellectual and emotional power, but your physical strength as well. Using a technique borrowed from Jack Canfield, president of Self-Esteem Seminars, she asks for volunteers to come to the front of the room and face the group. She then asks the volunteer to make a fist and hold her arm out with as much strength as she can muster. Jeffers then pushes down on the arm—never once, she says, has she been able to push down a participant's arm on the first try.

Then comes the interesting part. She instructs the volunteer to close her eyes and repeat ten times, "I am a weak and unworthy person." After the enervating statement has been repeated ten times, Jeffers asks her to extend her arm again, and to resist as hard as she can. "Immediately, I am able to bring down her arm. It is as though all her strength has left her," says Jeffers. Next, the volunteer is told to close her eyes and repeat ten times the positive statement, "I am a strong and worthy person." As expected, the arm then stays up when Jeffers tries to push it down. The message here is obvious: stop allowing your own negative thoughts to take away your emotional and physical power.[5]

Yet another form of negativity I see frequently is longing for the "good old days" and railing against the inevitable new forms. "We're waiting for the siege to end," Marjorie, a nurse in the day-surgery unit, told me. "We can't wait for this time of cost-cutting to be over, so we can go back to practicing the way we were trained." Marjorie had been a nurse for twenty years, and had watched disapprovingly as the hospital administration and the insurance industry seemed to put more and more emphasis on getting people in and out, rather than on delivering quality care. She belonged to a cadre of "good old days" complainers who gathered in the hospital snack bar at break time each morning, complaining about the heartless CEO, their ill-informed supervisors who they believed were forcing them to practice bad health care, and the government which was about to make it all worse.

Fortunately, Marjorie had a friend in pediatrics who had stopped going to the "bitch and moan" sessions, as she called them, because she believed they made things worse. She convinced Marjorie that her time would be better spent changing the negative energy than in spewing it around. "These are the new policies, and they're not going away," she told Marjorie, "so why don't we go to the hospital fitness room together tomorrow and ride the stationary bikes instead?" Marjorie tried it, was shocked at how different it made her feel, and never went back to the snack bar break. Instead, she and her friend rode their exercise bikes together and brainstormed ways to teach self-care to their patients and patients' caregivers, to make up for the shortened hospital stays. On her next performance evaluation, Marjorie's head nurse wrote, "Much improved attitude."

Do you find yourself longing for the good old days yourself, or working for someone who does, or supervising people who can't let go of the past? These are toxic-type situations; you'd best apply some of the antidotes described at the end of this chapter.

Recurrent Career Adversity Syndrome:
Yet Another Bad Break?

As we move away from our erroneous "I can't" beliefs, as
we build solid faith that we have within us the availability of
answers or guidance, we establish the mind-set needed for
life's true purposes.   —Marsha Sinetar

Recurrent Career Adversity Syndrome (RCAS) is a variation on
the theme of negativity. It's what I call the tendency to make the
same irrational interpretations of workplace situations again and
again, creating problems for you and your employer and keeping
you from being successful at your job. RCAS is tricky because it's
impossible to see in yourself unless someone points it out—at a
time when you've let down your defenses enough to take it in. Fritz,
for instance, was a public relations specialist who was referred to
me as part of an outplacement program when he was on his fourth
career crash in five years.

"I have the damnedest luck," he said when we first met. "I just
seem to run into one lousy organization after another."

RCAS is something every career counselor knows well, because
our offices are crammed full of people who have it, but who are often not about to admit to being any part of the problem. "Yes,
but . . ." is an RCAS sufferer's favorite phrase. The roots of RCAS
are often found in early traumas and disappointments. It can be
changed through one of two approaches: (1) by examining old unconscious memories and revising disabling "scripts," or (2) by a less
intrusive cognitive/behavioral therapy aimed at teaching different
ways of analyzing and coping with difficult situations. When career
counselors use a superficial approach, without either of these essential therapeutic change strategies as part of their tool kit, the results
can be disappointing for everyone.

There are five basic forms of RCAS but it's possible to have more
than one operational at any time. The five stances are the following:

- *The Generalizer:* "Everything is wrong now."
- *The Externalizer:* "Nothing is my fault."

- *The Internalizer:* "Everything is my fault."
- *The Personalizer:* "Why does everything happen to me?"
- *The Catastrophizer:* "This problem is too big to fix."

The Generalizer: "Everything Is Wrong Now."

Our friend Fritz, the public relations specialist, was a generalizer and an externalizer. He was blond, charming, good-looking, and in his early forties. He had a terrific sense of humor that enabled him to "interview well" and talk his way into situations. But time and time again, when problems occurred, Fritz's knee-jerk response was to blame someone else and then to create a story larger than the situation at hand.

"My last boss told me I was paranoid," Fritz boomed out in our first conversation. "Look who's calling who nuts. I'm never going to work for a guy like that again. I tried to tell him how other guys were screwing up the accounts so much that we were in danger of going under, but he just wouldn't listen." No wonder Fritz had found himself "on the list" when a merger required letting 10 percent of the staff go.

The Externalizer: "Nothing Is My Fault."

I asked Fritz to tell me about some of the other terrible work situations he'd experienced over the years. The litany was long and gruesome. And it was always somebody else's fault. It took several sessions for Fritz to tell me all the stories of abuse and stupidity he had endured at the hands of his employers. Eventually we got back to his college, and then his high school, experiences. True to form, his professors had been uninspiring—"a real disappointment considering how much it cost my parents to send me," he complained— and he was proud to say that he never gave any money to his college, just to let them know how dissatisfied he was.

Then came the big question. "And what can you tell me about your family life?" At first he was resistant. "I can't see what that has to do with anything," he countered. I could see myself about to be added to the list of stupid people he had encountered over the years, but I persevered. "Well, I think it may be relevant here, so just tell me a few situations and events you remember as important in your childhood and teen years. Then we can see if they're of any consequence."

Fritz, it turned out, was the oldest son of a career naval officer, who had often been away during Fritz's early years. He had four sisters and a brother, "each one conceived during a brief shore leave," he explained with a cynical twist to his mouth. His mother, overwhelmed by the demands of raising six children on her own, buoyed herself up with a combination of liquor and prescription drugs. Whenever his father returned home, there would be much yelling about her drinking and lack of organization, and Fritz would be called on to "shape things up around here and be the man of the house."

Is it any wonder that Fritz had carried around with him the assumption that things were always out of control? And didn't he long to be anyone but the person at fault with a family history like that? I asked him what positive things he had gotten from his upbringing. "Well, whenever my father came home we'd do a lot of entertaining to celebrate—he was a really social guy. I learned as a very little kid to talk to people, to be funny, and generally manage a party well."

And so there it was: the family had tutored him well in public relations skills, but it had also saddled him with the need to put any blame, which he found unbearable, on other people, and a feeling of being overwhelmed whenever things weren't as he thought they should be. In many ways he was still a ten-year-old struggling to make things OK in an out-of-control family situation.

At first Fritz thought my analysis was crazy: "shrink theory," he called it. But then I said I wouldn't be able to work with him unless he did some therapy at the same time, because I was convinced that the same troubles would recur in the next job unless he talked in more depth about some of that old material. He stormed away from that session. But after a month of turmoil and escalating bouts of digestive-tract symptoms, he finally called to ask if we could get together again to talk about what other steps he could take.

He agreed to do some short-term therapy through his HMO, and we kept working together. He found another job in a start-up public relations firm rather quickly, thanks to those old party skills of his, but he kept on with the therapy. It was a good thing, too, for it didn't take long in a brand-new organization, full of both promise and chaos, for Fritz's tendencies to show up. This time, however, the therapist helped him to talk about how nervous big risks made him, and to strategize how to break up large challenges into smaller, more manageable increments. When we last spoke things were going differently than in prior jobs.

The Internalizer: "Everything Is My Fault."

At the opposite end of the scale from Fritz's externalizing is Bobbie's internalizing stance. We began our session a few minutes late because I had been held up en route from a meeting. I arrived a little breathless to find Bobbie waiting in the reception area. "I'm so sorry to make you hurry" were the first words she said to me. *I was late, yet* she *was apologizing to* me *about it.*

Bobbie was an administrative assistant who had just been given an ultimatum from her boss: learn the computer applications we need you to know, learn the language and "style" of our customers, and move at a faster pace—or find work elsewhere. Bobbie was overwhelmed. "How can I be somebody I'm not?" she whined. Her feelings of desperation were made worse by the nearly constant lower back pain she endured. So I asked the RCAS question: "Has this ever happened before?"

It had, in a variety of settings, so that Bobbie was now convinced that perhaps she didn't belong anywhere. At first I considered that her current job might be just a poor fit, but then I asked her to tell me about the places she had worked where things were a little quieter, and where the style had matched hers a little better. Her response was telling.

"Well, it's like I think the job is going to fit me and then I get in there and I'm never quite right, no matter what they're expecting. It seems like I'm always disappointing somebody." Because Bobbie was all too willing to declare herself the problem, I didn't have to take the slow route as I had with Fritz. "Whom did you disappoint in your childhood?" I asked.

"How did you know? Almost everybody," she said quietly. Bobbie went on to describe being the youngest of four girls, and the one everybody had expected to be a boy, finally. When she turned out to be yet another girl, they named her Bobbie and decided that at least they could make her a tomboy. But Bobbie, who was small for her age, quiet, and absolutely uncoordinated, was boyish in name only.

She loved to read and draw, but hated the math and science that her engineer father tried to force on her. She had decided at an early age that the best way to stay out of trouble was to stay out of sight. School was never a good experience for her because she lived in dread of being called on. She decided not to go to college after high school because she didn't want to use up the family's resources.

And here she was now, in danger of being fired because she had spent a lifetime trying to be invisible. She had long mastered the art of calibrating her own energies and activities to be a few decibels below the norm for whichever situation she found herself in. So it wasn't a matter of fit for Bobbie. Until the basic problems of invisibility and her own feeling of worthlessness were addressed, the situation would continue to recur.

I suggested to Bobbie that she go shop first for a chiropractor and then for a therapist. It seemed important for her to "interview" several therapists and *choose* the one she liked. She did, and selected a woman about her own age with a personal style that seemed very similar to hers. Together they worked on both the concrete problems (where to get the computer training she needed) and the more elusive ones—how to be less invisible. Bobbie decided to tell her boss about the counseling, and to set some clear and explicit goals about how her performance would improve. Her boss was pleased with her new forthrightness, and things improved. The best part was that the job then felt new to Bobbie, who enjoyed feeling equal to what was being asked of her, perhaps for the first time in her life. What's more, as the tension in her body dissipated, and she worked on the exercises and stretches prescribed by the chiropractor, so did the disabling lower back pain.

The Personalizer: "Why Does Everything Happen to Me?"

Other manifestations of RCAS also present as "stuck again" situations. Personalizers get themselves in trouble in organizations, and hence are likely to be laid off or dismissed for cause, because they perceive normal conflicts and problems as personal assaults. The rebuke or the dismissal, then, becomes more fuel for their assumption that things are always being done to them.

Derek, a somewhat burly intense salesman in his early thirties, created a stir wherever he went. He carried around the potent memory of being one of the few students in his high school graduating class who didn't get to go to college. So he had decided to get even by making more money. In some ways, it was lucky he worked in outside sales, because the level of scrutiny on him was less there than had he spent all day with the same people. It was also easier to get new sales jobs after a parting of the ways. Derek's latest bout of personalization began when shipping mixed up the orders for his four biggest customers. Instead of working quickly with shipping and the sales manager to get the correct orders on their way, accompanied by an apologetic "we value your business" offering, Derek decided to take on the shipping manager. He accused him of deliberately sabotaging the shipments because he didn't like Derek. When the sales manager told Derek he thought he was off base, Derek took it as proof that people like him weren't wanted at that company. He pushed the sales manager for days to reconsider his disposition of the matter before he finally gave up. He told the head of shipping, "You won this time, but I've got my eye on you."

Derek came to counseling at the suggestion of the company employee assistance program specialist, who thought he deserved one last chance to deal with this personalizing pattern before being let go. Life in organizations is stressful enough, without allowing personalizers to contaminate the environment even more. Unlike Fritz and Bobbie, however, Derek wasn't willing to talk about RCAS, and so he was soon terminated—and on his way to another organization, convinced that people had treated him badly again.

The Catastrophizer: "This Problem Is Too Big to Fix."

Catastrophizers make themselves agitated (and often sick) by overreacting to setbacks. This proclivity hinders their ability to respond effectively to challenges. They often can't differentiate the essential from the secondary or can't mount a calm plan of action. Sometimes they come to me wanting to leave their current job because things seem so out of control, and sometimes they are helped out the door by a supervisor who's tired of responding to imagined crises.

Gary was a catastrophizer who got hysterical one too many times. A dispatcher for a small fleet of trucks, he found it hard not to get rattled when the calls piled up. When he had several problems needing responses, he would go into panic mode and call the boss, demanding to put one or more drivers on overtime to handle the overflow. He had just been let go because his supervisor felt he needed someone who could handle pressure better. When we talked about whether this tendency to seize up happened at home as well, Gary admitted that it did.

"My wife says I'm a control freak," he said. "I just seem to lose it when a problem looks overwhelming to me."

"So this is a problem you need to solve not only for your career, but for everybody's peace of mind at home also," I observed. He nodded somewhat sheepishly. And so we began a three-session program in which he learned to identify what triggered panic reactions for him, and to calm himself with a breathing exercise and visualization.

If you have RCAS, this is not a garden-variety "poor fit" we're talking about. It probably won't be fixed by finding another situation more to your liking. Rather, this is a consistent, recurrent pattern of taking the family laundry to work each day, no matter what the setting. Only liberal applications of self-awareness, preferably with some therapeutic detergent, will enable you to leave it at home.

Not only do Recurrent Career Adversity Syndrome sufferers cause themselves pain, but they make things difficult for co-workers too, filling work environments with tension and discord. They have an uncanny way of escalating minor adversity into major confrontations and luring coworkers into the toxic circle of conflict. If you're finding yourself frequently singed by office brushfires and wondering why, chances are you're working with one or more people afflicted with RCAS. The best advice for you: *get some distance,* and consider recommending one or more of the solutions in the next section.

Eight Great Escape Routes

The biggest sin is sitting on your ass.   —FLORYNCE KENNEDY

Perhaps the most important thing to be said about getting unstuck is that this is the time when you're required to say what you're for as well as what you're against. Much of the quagmire of being stuck has to do with negative, oppositional thinking:

- "I don't approve of how they treat people around here, so I don't put myself out for anybody."
- "I can't get a job I like because there's always an inside candidate."
- "What's the point in trying to get ahead when the company can fire you tomorrow?"
- "It's not my fault that nobody told me I'd need more education."
- "No, I'm not going to do any special preparations for that interview. I'm just going to be who I am."
- "I know I'm never gonna get promoted here because the boss doesn't like me, so there's not much use in trying."

Wallowing in angst about the unfairness of it all will compound the problems you're having, and have adverse health consequences as well. RCAS is a painful affliction. It keeps you locked in a constantly recurring pattern of agitation and dissatisfaction. People who find a way to break free feel jubilant about their escape. If you think you might be stuck in a pattern of recurrent career adversity, the only sensible thing to do is to declare war on your own negativity and *get help*. If you know someone else who is, you might want to find a way to talk a little about this book with him or her.

Remember the driveway, with the rivulets redesigning it each time it rained? Not until I took rake and shovel to it and flattened out those crevices did the water go the way I wanted it to. I would wager that many people are stuck in old patterns because they're following the path of least resistance. Only the structural changes of redesigning their assumptions (flattening those crevices) can help them move beyond that place. Here are some of the strategies that can be used:

- Bibliotherapy
- Back-to-school days
- Talk, talk, talk
- Escapee interviews
- Mental pictures
- Writing
- Brainwalking
- Going professional

With all these strategies, a *career log* is a very helpful companion. A looseleaf notebook, divided into sections keyed to whatever it is you're trying to accomplish, lets you collect your own feelings and thoughts, as well as information and suggestions you gather from other people. It's also a place to store relevant articles and reading notes. You design the sections as you go along, and the log becomes an important record of your journey. This is particularly important when you're wallowing in ambiguity, trying to decide whether to go, stay, or up-end your life. A record of your thoughts, feelings, and research helps you see that something really is happening.

Bibliotherapy

We seem to be a people who like to read about how to do things better. Career-related books and articles come in four quite different categories:

- *Self-assessment*—Books that show you how to get an honest reading on your interests, skills, values, and passions. They're important because work that doesn't fit who you really are will eventually make you ill.
- *Career information*—An inside look at various fields and functional areas.
- *Job search*—The nuts and bolts of cover letters, résumés, interviews, networking, and marketing yourself.
- *Career management*—How to play the game in different fields, how to position yourself for advancement, and what changes and developments to expect in your field over the next several years.

Each category is important, but the timing of when to consult each one is critical also. Reading about job search before you know what you're looking for can be confusing and anxiety-provoking. I always get "stuck" people into some self-assessment reading as the first step in turning around a problematic script of failure. Barbara Sher's book *I Could Do Anything I Want If Only I Knew What It Was* offers sensible and witty advice about getting going from a negative place.

Back-to-School Days

Perhaps you feel stuck because there are things you don't know and you doubt your ability to pick up new things. Maybe you need actual job skills, such as better computer training or a course in direct mail marketing. Or you might benefit from courses or seminars in topics such as strategic planning, writing, or effective communication. I've been delighted to see the proliferation of so many seminars and workshops in creative thinking over the past year or so, and so I often send people who have trouble imagining other options for themselves to some "mental gymnastics" training.

It's a safe bet that you need to be in some kind of educational situation on an ongoing basis. At Motorola, for instance, every employee is required to "go to school" at least one week of every year. If you're not sure what courses or workshops to be taking, ask your boss, a trusted co-worker, or a friend. Harvard Business School professor John Kotter, author of *The New Rules: How to Succeed in Today's Post-Corporate World,* has this to say about your need to keep on learning: "The person who attempts to coast, only applying what he or she has learned in the past, will have an increasingly difficult time being competitive in a tough global labor market. Economic forces will make the maxim GROW OR DIE."[6] If stepping off the path of least resistance has been hard for you, a well-chosen structured educational experience could be just the catalyst you need.

Talk, Talk, Talk

Talk is critical for getting out into the sunlight the moldy, self-limiting things you've been feeling and thinking. It will make your immune system happy, take some pressure off a muscle group or two, and probably even have a positive effect on your blood pressure. It can also get you firsthand information about other ways of handling whatever problems you're stuck in, about other resources for getting unstuck, or about other fields or organizations that may fit you. The emotional release would be worth it even if you didn't learn a single correct fact.

Hard as it may seem, you also need feedback. It's essential to know what others think of your skills and your approaches to situations in order to get moving out of a stuck place. I don't mean either brutal or sugar-coated feedback, so you need to choose your messengers carefully. Choose people who you know value you, who understand something about your general goals, who are able to be honest with you, and who are aware of their own issues and agendas. I'm sorry to say that significant others and family members, who often come with their own tangled relationship to you and your choices, are sometimes not the best resources.

This is a tough assignment, but here are some possible questions to spur conversations with others when trying to get extricated from a stuck place. Don't use them all at once—select the ones that seem most relevant.

Feedback for Breaking Out

The following questions are intended to shake things up a little, so don't be surprised if the answers make you feel a little off-center—that means the process of helping you to break out of your stuck places is working. Ask people you trust to give you honest responses to some of the following questions. During or after the conversation, record the ideas in your career log.

- What skills and talents have you seen me using well?
- What skills do you think I would need to develop more in order to be more effective in the work I'm doing?
- What other kinds of work could you imagine me doing well? Tell me why you think I'd be good at those jobs. (Ask for specific examples and skills.)
- What "stuck places" have you seen me get into? Do you have any observations about how I got myself there?
- What effective interpersonal strategies have you seen me use? What ineffective ones?
- What better methods of managing relationships could you suggest?
- What character strengths have you observed in me that might be useful now?
- What effective and ineffective problem-solving have you seen me do?

- Are there resources you or other people have found helpful from which you think I could benefit?

Be sure to keep a record of what people say in your career log, so that you can look back over the information for consistent responses that resonate. It's also important to write it down because people forget more than 90 percent of what they hear within a month. This "golden" feedback is too precious to lose. Piloting a career at any level without honest feedback is the equivalent of dismissing all the air traffic controllers at the airport. But still people resist it: you might find more enthusiasm for regular root-canal procedures.

In organizations, you often get the most helpful feedback by querying your boss, your peers, and your direct reports about your effectiveness, and comparing your perceptions to theirs. This process is called 360-degree feedback. If you work in a large organization, ask whether the human resources department offers this service. People in smaller settings can contact career consultants individually about this kind of intensive feedback.

Escapee Interviews

Almost everybody these days knows somebody who successfully got out of some kind of career trap. In your career log, make a list of every escapee you and the people you know can think of, with a notation about what kind of trap they managed to break free of. When the list has at least ten names on it, order them according to whose story grabs you the most and set up a time to interview that person. Ask the escapee what he or she did, how long it took to plan, what doubts had to be overcome, anything else that might be helpful. Don't worry about imposing. Given the numbers of toxic workplaces, you are in a long line of people waiting to break out, and someday you'll be willing to be interviewed by another escapee-in-the-making. After your first interview, work your way down the list, taking careful notes in your career log after each conversation. You'll be surprised what a jump-start this modeling exercise (as in showing you how it's done) can give your own campaign.

Mental Pictures

Visualizing desired behaviors and goals is a critical skill that most performance consultants spend lots of time teaching their clients. Various approaches to visualizing desired outcomes, such as neurolinguistic programming (NLP) and a technique called "Triggers,"[7] are available. "Stimulus Management" technologies allow you to make irritating or frustrating situations more bearable. Similarly, visualization tools let you train your mind to respond positively rather than negatively to challenges or crises. Because of the tremendous power of your beliefs in enhancing or limiting your behavior, visualizing being unstuck and on your way to someplace is a critical first step.

The second step, then, is to practice in your brain getting where you want to be. This is possible because your body can't really distinguish between actual physical practice and visualized practice: a blend of the two will get the best result. Mental pictures were helpful to Charlene, a social worker whose talents and passions were obscured by her aversion to risk.

When she arrived for counseling, Charlene let me know that she needed a change, but that the process just seemed overwhelming. She had been a social worker for more than twenty years, and had actively disliked it for at least fifteen of them. By the time she got to me, she was being treated for lupus erythematosis, an autoimmune disease, and considering early retirement and partial disability.

Charlene had always been cautious. Her mother had told her that she didn't walk alone until she was almost two, and for most of her life she had chosen to perpetuate the view of herself as a careful person who didn't take silly risks. Fortunately, during the time that she was seeing me, Charlene was assigned a new client at her agency, a young woman who also had chronic illness and who was choosing to sit by and let life happen to her. This young woman presented Charlene with such an inescapable reflection of herself that she had no choice but to confront her own passivity (another bucket in the hallway).

Fluent in Spanish and an avid reader, Charlene analyzed her interests and was surprised to discover that she could really get excited about one-on-one teaching or tutoring. After a period of some consideration, she decided she might like to teach adult literacy and English as a second language classes. That decided, the next step was to work on Charlene's risk-taking skills. I asked her to do some "internal investigation" in a guided-imagery exercise, to make contact with the part of her that was afraid of implementing this new plan. She found that she had internalized her mother's fear that if someone lost a job, there would be no other opportunities for work. She knew that her mother's childhood had been shadowed by her own father's inability to find a job after his was lost during the Depression. So the risk-aversive self inside Charlene was trying to protect her from a loss similar to her grandfather's.

I asked her next to call on her internal "creative self" to come up with three ways to make the change she was considering safer. After hesitating and then stumbling a little, Charlene finally got her logical, fearful self out of the way and let her more positive, intuitive self generate three different possibilities:

- Doing some more reading and informational interviewing, to learn about other people who changed their work and lived to tell about it.
- Joining a career support group.
- Asking her boss for a partial change in her assignment on a pilot basis, in case she didn't like the new work.

"Those are great ideas," I told her. "Which ones do you think you'd like to try?" Charlene decided to do all three, in that order. In a few weeks, she was ready to think about approaching the director of her agency to propose cutting her work to part-time in order to do an internal apprenticeship, offering language classes and tutoring to Spanish-speaking clients. If the program seemed useful, she would suggest that they renegotiate her contract for the next year to include language instruction.

She was terrified about making such a request, so to prepare for asking her boss, she invited a co-worker with knowledge of the boss's style and likely reactions over to dinner. After a relaxing meal, they used a tape recorder and actually practiced various ways the conversation might go.

The next day Charlene listened to the tape, chose the scenario she liked best, and wrote a script for her approach to the boss. Then she put herself on a "dry run" schedule for the next week, rehearsing her speech in the car every day during the thirty-minute ride to work. She also made a mental image of herself actually doing the language classes and the tutoring that she intended to ask the boss permission to do. This all might seem elementary to some seasoned risk takers, but Charlene had an old, stubborn pattern of caution and obedience from which to extricate herself. By the time the day for her meeting with the boss came, she was convinced she'd get what she was asking for—and she did. Even if risk-taking comes easier to you than it did to Charlene, there's no harm in doing practice visualizations—even Olympic athletes use them, after all. In the competitive, toxic places where you're trying to succeed, you need all the practice you can get.

You can also use visualization to overcome the unfortunate but natural resistance that most stuck people come to feel about climbing out of their own particular swamp. Here are some of the visualized successes I've seen. Jim got himself out of a depressing sales slump by recalling the thrill of playing Curly in his high school rendition of *Oklahoma!* just before sales calls. Meg prepared for successfully negotiating a four-day week for herself by revisualizing her best season on the debate team in college. Laura tapped into the power she needed to fire a "toxic" subordinate by recalling a successful sales presentation with a difficult customer. And Todd practiced convincing his boss to send him to an expensive executive development program by revisualizing winning the soccer championship his senior year in college.

In situations like these, you pair a remembered positive stimulus with the thing you're trying to do, in order to overcome your fear. When working with people who are about to have frightening job interviews or to ask for something they want at work, for instance, I teach them how to charge an imaginary battery with the power they'll need to present themselves in an engaging and energetic way. Here's how the visualization goes:

> First choose some accessible spot on your body that you will use as an "anchor"—a place which, when you touch it, can call to mind the qualities and emotions you want available to you. Good choices might be on the back of your hand (not the palm), your wrist, or your arm—a spot you can remember and reach easily no matter what position your body is in, and which doesn't have a lot of other associations connected with it. Rest the fingers of your free hand lightly on that place as you continue with the exercise.
>
> Sit comfortably, close your eyes, and remember a time when you were very pleased with an accomplishment. Recall a situation when you knew you had done something well, and you felt like a real winner. Remember what was going on all around you—where you were, who else was there, what was happening. What sounds, smells, sights, and especially feelings, can you remember? See it with your eyes, hear it, sense it as if you are living it *right now.*
>
> When you feel the scene is intensely real, apply pressure with your fingers on the spot you have chosen for about a count of six. Then open your eyes and distract yourself for a moment. Close your eyes again and return to the scene of your accomplishment. Repeat the steps above, trying to make it even more vivid than it was last time. When you feel that you are at the height of your being "present" in that moment, press your "anchor" (or "trigger"—another name for the same phenomenon) again and hold it for a count of six. To make absolutely sure you have it, do it one more time, again working to make the memory even more a "present-time event."
>
> When it comes time for the interview (or any other situation when you need to be maximally ready for a challenge), just press your spot. The recall of that positive memory, with all the same positive emotions, will just come to you, and all the "power" you need will be at your disposal.

Writing

Writing can pull you out of stuck places. It lets you record what's going on for you, as well as information you collect, which can be useful at decision-making times. Getting unstuck often requires the kind of cleaning out that is best done with a pen or computer. Writing things down also shows that you take the whole process seriously, which is an important part of breaking free. In order to get some of the important things up from your unconscious and out where you can look at them, here are some questions to respond to, not just once, but on a regular basis. Collect your answers to the following in your career log.

- What strengths do I know I have?
- What limitations am I trying to overcome?
- What childhood experiences might have been responsible for writing the "script" of my strengths and limitations?
- What fears get in my way when I think of really succeeding at work I love? What might be the sources of those fears?
- What negative beliefs about myself have I allowed to get in my way? Where did those beliefs come from?
- How much do I believe that I deserve to have work I love? If not, why not?
- How might my parents' own career "dramas" be influencing the places where I'm stuck right now?
- What might the "costs" be, to my relationships and to the way my life is currently arranged, if I were to get unstuck? What would have to change? Am I willing to take those risks?

If the questions are new to you and this seems like a dumb exercise, that's all the more reason to do it. Perhaps there's some comfort in the findings of university researchers that when students write about previously held-back problems, they experience improved immune functioning. This is consistent with other research reported throughout the book that "unloading" feelings is associated with better rates of recovery from all kinds of disease.

Brainwalking

Like brainstorming, brainwalking is about moving beyond stale paradigms and generating creative solutions to problems. The physical activity jars loose many more ideas about how to get unstuck than you'd get sitting in a chair. The best effects come from doing your brainwalking outside, where Nature can work her healing on you at the same time. But if you're a city dweller or if it's icy and wet outside, you can get in some good "breaking free" steps in a mall, at an indoor track, or by walking briskly through public buildings. You can even do it on your own treadmill, so long as you're careful not to lose your footing during the jotting-down-notes part.

Before you begin your walk, focus intently on an obstacle that seems to be keeping you stuck, and tell your unconscious that you'd like some fresh new ways to get around this obstacle. Carry with you a "think pad" of some sort (I use ten or so index cards, but can also recommend a small spiral notebook) and a felt-tip pen. I've found that twenty to thirty minutes is a good amount of time for generating jailbreak ideas. As you carry your focused question into your brainwalk, the ideas begin to pop just like those little colored balls in the Fisher-Price popper toys. That's why you have a felt-tip pen in hand—to stop momentarily and jot down ideas that come. This is called "harvesting." I've learned the hard way that ideas which come to you in this intense walk-think mode are excellent but evanescent. If you don't capture them as they erupt, you won't remember most of them at the end of the walk. Another great thing about brainwalking for busy people is that it's efficient. You get to exercise your intellect, your muscles, and your cardiovascular system all at the same time.

Going Professional

Unfortunately, there are afoot in our individualistic work culture strong biases against seeming vulnerable, which might be keeping you from getting the professional "unloading" help you need to turn problematic situations into major growth events. Because those prejudices run wide and deep, I'm assuming that some readers will not avail themselves of the professional help that could make a tremendous difference. For them, this book and the array of other resources available in bookstores and workshop programs will have to suffice. Hopefully, no one will give up on the situation altogether.

Career counselors are obviously the first line of helpers you might consider in looking for someone to help you put workplace toxicity in perspective. Career counselors can be found in private practice, of course, but also in such places as colleges, libraries, women's centers, adult education centers, community health organizations, HMOs, and special agencies such as Alumnae Resources in San Francisco and the Women's Educational and Industrial Exchange in Boston.

Choosing carefully is as much a concern when selecting a career counselor as when purchasing anything else; it's important to be an informed consumer. Among the qualities that anyone you'd consider seeing should possess are the following:

- Training in counseling skills as well as in various self-assessment techniques; preferably an advanced degree and licensing or certification by a recognized board or agency.
- Access to useful and updated workplace information—in the office or nearby.
- Recent experience with "real" employers.
- A policy of confidentiality and experience in making referrals to therapists or physicians, should you experience emotional or physical difficulties during the career-exploration process.
- The ability to interpret frequently used assessment instruments, such as the Myers-Briggs Type Inventory (MBTI), interest surveys, intelligence tests, aptitude profiles such as the Johnson O'Connor System, and learning-style inventories.
- A reasonable, flexible price structure without requirements to purchase an expensive "package" of services up front, before it's clear just what your needs are going to be.
- A commitment to career counseling as a service to individuals rather than just a series of products for sale.

Don't be shy about asking questions. When you find someone who meets most of the above criteria, chances are you'll be in reliable hands.

A psychotherapist can also be a career explorer's best ally. There's no point in going through the pain of a career upheaval if you don't get some good growth out of it. A career crisis is not meant to be fixed and forgotten. Quite the contrary, the purpose is to learn something about yourself, for use in both your personal and professional life. Being alive is about learning and growing: many of your best lessons will occur at work if you're alert enough to study them. Being stuck should be a very bright red flag for you to stop and ask what learning there is that has been trying unsuccessfully to happen.

Therapy comes in many styles. The simplest is probably a brief therapy regime available for anywhere from five to fifteen sessions through your HMO. Now that the medical profession is reading evidence that brief therapy can reduce stress-related medical problems by as much as 50 percent, many of you may find yourselves referred more frequently to the mental health side of the house.

Of course there are more extensive forms of therapy that are quite helpful as well. Traditional psychodynamic individual work is perhaps the most intense way to excise emotional malignancies that are getting in your way at work. Groups are also quite effective, as they offer a chance for feedback from more than one person and an arena to "practice" better ways of handling workplace stumbling blocks and dilemmas.

Other therapies (some more practical and strategic, others more spiritual) can also help you unravel the conscious and unconscious threads of workplace dilemmas. Neurolinguistic programming, hypnotherapy, transactional analysis, focusing, cognitive/behavioral approaches, psychosynthesis, biofeedback, expressive therapies, movement therapy, body-mind centering, Rolfing, and shamanic counseling are all part of the potpourri. What's available and who's good in your location is something you'll have to discover for yourself by asking around or calling a local referral service.

There's no doubt that psychotherapy heals—not only emotionally, but physically. Studies of recovering cancer, heart disease, arthritis, asthma, and skin-disorder patients have shown repeatedly, for instance, that support groups and individual psychotherapy seem to enhance the effectiveness of other treatments. Research by major corporations into the relationship between psychotherapy and the physical health of their employees has shown up to an 85 percent decrease in health-care utilization costs for people who choose to talk about what's bothering them at work. In another pilot study in Hawaii, utilization of medical and surgical care decreased by half for patients who took advantage of brief psychotherapy. Having employees take a closer look at what they're feeling might be more palatable if employers knew it could save them fifty cents on the dollar.

Much of the research on the efficacy of therapy says that it doesn't matter which modality you choose, so long as you commit to using whatever career dysfunction you're feeling as an imperative to dig deeper into what work means to you in the context of your whole life. If you choose someone you believe in, because she or he has been recommended and because your intuition tells you it's a good fit, then the style won't make much difference.

And don't forget about your physician. "I treat lots of sprained careers," one family practitioner told me during an interview. Physicians are very helpful in designing ways to be treating your body better, and they are also a ready resource to consult about whether some medication might be helpful. Gary, the catastrophizing dispatcher and husband, for instance, found that habit a lot easier to kick after he got some help from low doses of an anti-anxiety drug.

Going It Alone or with Help: Just Get Going!

If you aren't fired with enthusiasm, you will be fired with enthusiasm. —VINCE LOMBARDI

People who are stuck need to do something, almost anything, to overcome the inertia they've been feeling. The famous composer and music critic Virgil Thomson said, "Try a thing you haven't tried before three times—once to get over the fear, once to find out how to do it, and a third time to find out whether you like it or not." Try any one of the resources suggested in these chapters. If the first one doesn't work, try another one, until you get the engine of change to turn over a time or two. Then you'll be ready for the next chapters on how to revitalize a tired career or create a more energizing fit between you and work.

5. Revitalizing Your Career

If in the last few years you haven't discarded a major opinion or acquired a new one, check your pulse. You may be dead. —GELETT BURGESS

Even if you're not stuck, you need to shake things up in your career from time to time. It's often a lot more trouble to figure out what's not working quite so well anymore than to go along with the established routine. But when you ignore your dissatisfactions, you wear down your resistance without even knowing it, until your body wakes you up with a "symptom"—some kind of pain or disease. Even if you aren't "stuck" in the negative ways we discussed in Chapter 4, you need to keep your work "new," in one way or another, in order to stay healthy.

Sometimes the problem is that others close to you are pressuring you to keep up the status quo. Take Liz's situation. A gregarious single woman in her mid-thirties, she came to me feeling atrophied in her position with a major insurance company. Her uncle had gotten her a job with the company a decade ago, and she had risen through the ranks from underwriter to regional sales manager. At first she had liked the work. Despite her success, however, as things had gotten tighter at the company, it just wasn't much fun anymore. Liz was itching to try something different. Yet she felt paralyzed, because every time she even hinted about leaving her job, a litany of responsibility from her mother pelted her: "What do you mean you're not satisfied with your job? I worked twenty-three years for the same company and never missed a day, just to put food on the table for you kids after your father left us. Do you think I did that for fun? When are you ever going to grow up?"

Liz had finally come to my office on the suggestion of her doctor, who was treating her for migraines. When Liz and I first met, she was feeling pretty down on herself, wondering why the money and responsibility in her current job weren't enough to make her want to stay. I asked Liz some standard questions, such as what she liked to do in her spare time, what achievements she remembered from her early years as being really fun, and what made her feel good about herself. I made a list as she talked.

Most of the items on Liz's current list had very little to do with the insurance business. "My list would have looked different ten years ago," she remarked. "I really loved doing sales when I started out." But now she was an avid reader who liked nothing better than to haunt old bookstores. She was a gourmet cook. She also enjoyed being with people, even though she had allowed her social life to dwindle over the past several years as her work had become more and more toxic for her. As a child and adolescent, she had also been a risk-taker, pushing herself in athletic events and contests of various sorts. But now she felt too beaten down to be doing anything risky.

We worked together with her list for several sessions, helping her to recall old passions and considering how the greatest number of the things she really enjoyed might come together in a new way. She decided to draw one of her friends, who was also aching to leave her job, into the scheme. Slowly a shape emerged: they decided they would like to open a small bookstore cafe. Once Liz felt that she was on her way out of the insurance industry, her stress level abated. Next came the plan.

Liz decided she would work part-time in a bookstore on weekends and attend some seminars on starting and running a business. Her friend Susan would do the same thing on the restaurant side of the business. They would also take advantage of free consultations at the Small Business Administration. They would create the actual business plan gradually, as they learned things both firsthand and from their seminars.

Liz agreed to put some energy back into her life by reviving some of her social connections. She also promised to pay more attention to her health generally: if she continued to starve herself of fun, exercise, and good nutrition, she'd never have the vitality to pull off the changes she and Susan were planning. Within eighteen months, they had firmed up a business plan, and Liz said good-bye to her migraines. Even her mother had to admit the change was a good one. Liz and Susan were reassured by the statistic that the millions of jobs lost in Fortune 500 downsizings had been created anew in women-owned businesses. They had also done a great deal of homework, including intensive market research, and were confident that the combination of books, cards, prints, and a cafe atmosphere could succeed in their college town. As we were ending our last session, Liz reminded me of one of her favorite Corita Kent lines: "Flowers grow out of dark moments." Indeed they had for Liz.

In analyzing a toxic-work situation, an important piece of the puzzle is how long people have been doing the same work without significant changes and opportunities for growth. Liz's headaches forced her to confront what she didn't really want to know—partly because change is always at least somewhat unsettling, and partly because it meant inviting her mother's and uncle's disapproval.

In Liz's and other clients' stories over the years, I've found an interesting pattern. The image that has emerged is a bell-shaped curve of how people relate to their work over time. In most instances there appear to be five stages through which we all progress. The first four stages are virtually inevitable: Stage 1, Getting started; Stage 2, Getting better; Stage 3, Peak performance; and Stage 4, in which you feel that "Something is missing." But Stage 5, in which your relation to your work is in major trouble, isn't. This is yet another choice point.

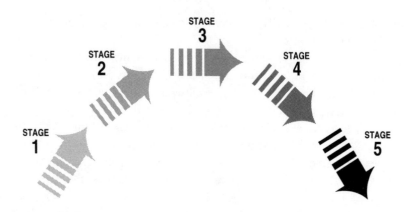

Stage 1—Getting started. High energy, but some mistakes. Strong optimism paired with strong anxiety.

Stage 2—Getting better. Less frenetic energy, fewer mistakes. More focus and efficiency. Feeling more confident all the time.

Stage 3—Peak performance. Things are really going well. Surely this can last forever!

Stage 4—"Something is missing." Lower energy, less personal investment and reward. Frustration, boredom, disappointment.

Stage 5—Major trouble. Impaired self-esteem, stress, physical symptoms. Time to change the way you're doing your job or prepare to leave.

Here's how the stages work. Predictably, as you begin any new job or work assignment (Stage 1), you journey up the hill from start-up excitement, to getting better (Stage 2), to peak experience and effectiveness (Stage 3). At the top of the bell-shaped curve, you feel as if your success will last forever. Or will it? Most people climb up to the crest of the mountain, stay poised there awhile, and then start the descent into a state of minor dissatisfaction (Stage 4).

There is very little hint as you reach the peak experience of Stage 3 that you will be required to navigate your way down the other side, at least not until it's happened a few times. On the way down, unfortunately, you find yourself sliding first into disappointment and moodiness. If you don't do something to slow down or reverse the downward movement, such as learning new skills or arranging to do some aspect of your work differently, then disillusionment, sadness, anger, and illness (Stage 5) are not far behind.

People usually ask, "Is this inevitable? Do I have to plummet to Stage 5?" Not at all, when you expect the inevitable changes ("Shifts happen!") and learn to manage them. When you find yourself entering a Stage 4 period, you have three choices:

- Dead work
- New work
- Revitalized work

Dead work happens when you've been at your job too long, without varying some parts of what you're doing or learning enough new things. The obvious down side of dead work is the emotional and physical discomfort that follows. For employers, the problem is the diminution of worker productivity and creativity, at a time when they've never been needed more.

New work is what happens when you decide to change jobs altogether to escape Stages 4 and 5. Your work becomes new and exciting again, as you start over at Stage 1. The down side of new work is that you may have to leave valued friends and colleagues. You may also give up some of the "reputation points" you've earned with your current employer. And there is a strong likelihood of losing ground financially rather than gaining it. According to one study, in the early nineties only about one in five people who changed jobs moved to a position making more money. For employers, the down side is that someone has to start from the beginning in two places to train new workers, adding a cost of 50 percent or more to each new worker's first-year salary.

But *revitalized work* interrupts that slide into the depths of Stage 5. When you reach Stage 4, you move back over to Stage 2 and the positive side of the curve. Workers and supervisors collaborate to build new tasks and learning opportunities into their jobs by redefining and redistributing assignments. You're able to be renewed and challenged, and yet stay within the same work unit. It's a win-win all around. You get to stay with the organization where you have benefits, seniority, and important relationships, while your employer keeps essential employees and saves on hiring and retraining costs. Your employer also has an opportunity to move people laterally as part of a "broad-band" approach to deploying staff. What is the cost for this miracle program? Not very much. For you, it costs your willingness to be flexible, imaginative, and assertive, for you'll probably have to be the one to start the process. For your boss, the costs include some training in listening skills and innovation facilitation. It's a very good deal all round.

You may find yourself working in a situation where your career revitalization needs are not much of a priority for the folks in charge. That usually means leaving—but you'll want to do it on your own schedule. An effective tool for lengthening your tether is a previously discussed technology called neurolinguistic programming (NLP). Using NLP lets you have a choice about what you're experiencing. By learning to manipulate the size and intensity of the stimuli you encounter, you can "reprogram" yourself to be less affected by people and situations you find distasteful.

Marilyn, for instance, was pushed over into Stage 4 by the arrival of a supervisor whose style could not have been more different from her own. Marilyn was very orderly and structured in her approach to work, preferring to stick with one task until she had finished it satisfactorily. But her boss, Sylvia, who had been left with two units to pull together in the aftermath of a downsizing, had more than she could handle. Sylvia's desk was piled high with projects in varying stages of completion, and she was not interested in discussing her style with anyone or in giving her staff permission to alter their jobs. (So much for "revitalized work" for Marilyn.)

Marilyn knew she couldn't stay long in this restructured organization with this overloaded manager, but she had no place to go at that point in time. To lessen the strain, she learned to approach the boss's desk as if she were filming it, making a video in her brain. She distanced from the chaos by imagining that she could adjust the lens for much longer distance shots, and dim the light as well. Hence the pile, which had come to her to symbolize an unsafe organization, with no one really in charge, was a long way away, hidden in shadows, and much less menacing. This simple manipulation of mental images enabled Marilyn to feel calmer and less at risk at work each day, while she searched for a job reporting to a manager whose style and workload were more comfortable for her. (On to "new work" for Marilyn.)

Others needing a change but wanting to buy some time have chosen to "turn down the volume" or "change the colors" on their imaginary TV. The end result is of course the same. When you make a choice to "manage" the sounds or sights until their emotional hold over you is diminished, you are free of the negative feelings for the moment. And when you've repeated the process often enough, the upsetting feelings don't come up as frequently or with the same intensity. You can then concentrate on making the changes you need to make without magnifying and obsessing about the current annoyance.

Here are some other ways of staying connected while you search for "new work" that have worked for other people:

- If you're feeling unable to connect with the organization where you work in a positive way, focus on your field. You can rekindle interest in a professional group or subscribe to journals or trade magazines, independent of your feelings about your current employer.
- Focus your attention on individuals you admire in the organization or in your field. Let your desire to work with or learn from those people motivate you now.
- If you feel positive about the mission of the organization but not about the organization itself, see your work as a way of supporting the overall mission, even though you may disapprove of some of the practices. You can focus on the larger goals and, at least for the moment, blur out the details that bother you. I've seen organizations change in response to feedback from employees during times of upheaval so that the employees found they didn't have to leave after all. Whether you're going or finding a way back to Stage 2, however, you

have everything to gain from doing what it takes not to feel under siege and compromise your health while you're there.

- Concentrate on the camaraderie, looking forward to your time with your co-workers each day as the primary reason for going to work.

- Fix your attention on the skills you're trying to build or enhance to take with you to your next assignment, job, or career. Let training or practice in those areas sustain your interest.

This list probably seems like a hodgepodge of different strategies. It is—because people's personal styles and work motivations differ so. Do whatever works for you. The one thing you cannot afford to do is give up and lapse into helpless, complaining Stage 5 mode. Being committed to *something* about your work prolongs your ability to stay working and increases the likelihood that you'll remain healthy and energized while planning impending moves in or out of the organization. It also gives you time to search, which is critical now that strategic job moves are often taking six months to two years to pull off. Leaving in a huff and having to take the first thing that comes along just to keep the bill collectors at bay is hardly a health-enhancer.

Self-Esteem: Don't Let It Get Away!

When self-confidence becomes eroded, it just makes it harder to solve any other problems that come along. Our doubts about our own abilities become self-fulfilling prophecies . . . and then we forget we have created these boundaries ourselves.   —Jon Kabat-Zinn

The first three stages build your confidence; the other two take it away. As Stage 3 peaks and then slides into Stage 4, the creeping self-doubt will be barely perceptible if you're not expecting it. If you ignore the warning signals of Stage 4, however, you'll eventually find yourself in full-fledged Stage 5. Then your self-esteem falls away in chunks, leaving you nauseated or in pain on Monday mornings, depressed, and without the energy you need to make those changes that should have been made months or years before. It's a vicious cycle. You lose interest in your work and so you don't do it quite as well. Or perhaps the plunge speeds up when a new boss or a new set of tasks enters the scene—what used to be easy is now hard. Here's the most insidious scenario: you begin to question whether you'll be able to do it well, and your performance matches your expectations. Unless you consciously intervene and correct the expectation, your performance spirals downward and your self-esteem plummets. That's why a career crisis is often a great catalyst for wrestling with old self-esteem problems. There are many ways to attack the problem. Individual or group counseling is usually available through your health plan. You might also consider some of the interventions from Chapter 4.

But how hard is it to stay out of advanced Stages 4 and 5? That depends on how you talk to yourself. When your internal chatter is negative and self-doubting, getting going from Stage 4 back over to Stage 2 seems onerous. You just don't have the energy to be proactive. But when you feel relatively confident, and when you have good support systems in place, the flow is smoother. Individuals also bring different "psychological metabolism" to the process. Some move through the stages slowly, while others seem to zip up across and over at a brisker pace. The circular revitalizing motion—up, down, and then back across to Stage 2—can happen again and again with the same employer, when employees and their managers know what's happening and are willing to tinker with new "arrangements."

Up and Down the Mountain

Real development is not leaving things behind, as on a road, but drawing life from them, as from a root.
—G. K. CHESTERTON

Undulations in career enthusiasm and self-esteem were part of what brought Mark to my office. Mark was a tall, bearded thirty-year-old who took a major leap and traded in his on again–off again work as a carpenter and sometime wilderness guide to begin a new career as a worksite supervisor for juvenile offenders. Some of his old friends were baffled; this was a side of Mark they hadn't seen. Others saw the connection right away. The organizational parts of the job were tough for Mark at first, but he found it easy to talk to the students, who reminded him of himself as a teenager. He loved going to work each morning. His enthusiasm sustained him through many trying but important learning experiences (Stage 1) as he mastered the flow of paperwork and appointments.

Gradually he got better at combining what he knew of the trades and outdoor activities with his ability to communicate in clear and no-nonsense ways. The teenagers assigned to his work groups began to do very well at their jobs, and he got more and more positive feedback (Stage 2). Four years into this new career, he was sitting on top of the world, with really good results from his worker-students and a promotion to area training manager. He figured he had really found his niche (Stage 3).

But after a while his enthusiasm began to wane. Mornings didn't feel quite the same. His allergies flared up for the first time in years. Initially, he blamed it on his wife Alice's pregnancy and the stress of preparing for parenthood: he just had more to worry about now, he figured (enter Stage 4). His supervisor noticed the change in his energy level and suggested to Mark that he take a course in supervisory skills at the local university. There he could meet other managers from businesses and nonprofit organizations. That would also help him with motivating and evaluating the site supervisors who reported to him now. He took the course, made some great new friends in the field, and his enthusiasm was renewed (back to Stage 2).

Two years later, however, Mark found himself feeling itchy again. This time he was really hard on himself. "What's the matter with you? You have a managerial position with benefits, retirement, free tuition for courses, and a boss who likes you—all the stuff you thought you wanted. And now you think you're tired of it? Maybe you'll never really amount to anything after all."

So Mark tried harder at doing the same old things. But the more he tried, the worse he felt. An old back ailment flared up, and he had to miss work for several days. Still he kept pushing himself. Then he found himself immobilized for two weeks. Fortunately, Alice deduced what was going on. She had traveled a convoluted career path herself, from VISTA volunteer to artist to teacher. She saw his physical symptoms as evidence that he was trying unsuccessfully to apply the brakes on a natural evolutionary process. It was clear to her that Mark's pains and his depression were a sign to get moving and start the bell-shaped-curve process all over again. Here was the question: could it be back to Stage 2 for another retooling or should it be to Stage 1 someplace else? That's when Mark came to see me.

After much discussion and vacillation, Mark decided that he was glad about the somewhat unorthodox direction his career had taken, but that he really wanted a chance to make more money now. The security of a government-funded human services position had been an improvement over the uncertainty of a solo carpentry business. He had also enjoyed feeling that his work made a difference in kids' lives. But he was a parent himself now, and he wanted the challenge of having his earnings reflect the time and ingenuity he put into his work. He knew money would never be the be-all and end-all for him, but it was a factor he wanted to pay attention to at this point in his life. In his current organization, the salary structure was fair and consistent, but far below what he could make in business.

So Mark gathered up his courage and talked to his supervisor one April morning. He said how sorry he was, but he really felt that this time he had to leave. The supervisor had been through career shifts himself and understood. He was able to arrange for a gradual disengagement, one that would give Mark until fall to look for other things. He would be able to separate gradually from the kids and the other supervisors he was managing, who had gotten very attached to him. Mark was also glad to be able to help his supervisor by participating in hiring and training a new manager.

Then something amazing happened. Once Mark knew he was leaving and exploring new possibilities, his back pain went away and his enthusiasm returned. He had a terrific last several months on the job, and was able to leave feeling happy about his years there. Plotting his next moves didn't turn out to be so hard either. He combined his skills as a tradesman with the management skills he had been developing and joined forces with several other people he knew to start a home-improvement collaborative. The timing was right, and he was confident that there was good money to be made.

Of course his old friends teased him about going back to what seemed in some ways just like what he had left. But he was able to say with conviction that his new plan was quite different from his days as a solo carpenter. He was clear that his experience of counseling the teenagers assigned to him and then supervising other instructors had forced him to develop the maturity and reliability he'd need for this step. He was ready for this venture now in ways that he could not even have imagined before had all these episodes in his life not come together. Mark also assumed that his new business partnership would have its evolutionary stages as well. This time, however, he'll be better prepared to manage Stage 4 when it begins to happen.

Diagnosis: Burnout or Rustout?

One of the saddest things is that the only thing a man can do for eight hours a day, day after day, is work. You can't eat eight hours a day nor drink for eight hours a day nor make love for eight hours—all you can do for eight hours is work. Which is the reason why man makes himself and everybody else so miserable and unhappy.   —WILLIAM FAULKNER

When you find yourself slipping into Stage 4, it's difficult to know just where the problem lies. You need to give some hard thought to how long you've been in the same position and to whether what you're *required* to do still fits what you *want* to do. It's hard at first to differentiate burnout from rustout. Burnout happens when the stresses are too strong and the rewards too few, and some of your old baggage is getting in the way.

Sometimes the causes are external to you—oppressive managers, increased demands, or too little opportunity for autonomy. But it's likely that you have a hand in the problem yourself. Perhaps the overload is about your need to please or be liked, keeping you from setting clearer boundaries at work, even though it would be perfectly acceptable to do so. If you have a tendency toward burnout, *"Let me think about it and get back to you"* are ten life-saving words you need to use often. Burnout often results from a neurotic compulsion to give it all away.

Paul, a brand manager for a consumer products firm, was referred to me by his doctor. The open-ended nature of his job seemed to serve him up a never-ending supply of crises. The situation was worsened by his tendency to dream up more and more promotional schemes—just to be sure he was really doing a bang-up job. When we talked about a typical day at work, he asked me if I had seen that old *I Love Lucy* TV show episode in which Lucy and Ethel were boxing candies in a factory and just couldn't keep up with the chocolates coming by on the conveyor belt, no matter how hard they tried.

"That's what I feel like most of the time," he said. "I'm stuffing those chocolates into every hiding place I can find, and still they keep on coming." "And what do you think this has to do with your health?" I asked. "Well, whenever the conveyor belt really gets overloaded and I'm forced to put in one of my killer weeks, that's when I seem to get sick again."

For years, Paul had been uncomfortable with his pattern of being perpetually exhausted and broke. He knew he had repeatedly expanded the scope of his job just enough to be on the verge of not getting it all done. He also had a habit of extending himself financially just a little beyond his means, whatever those means were at the moment. It was as if a computer had programmed him to be 10 percent overexpended in both time and money, no matter where he worked or what he was earning. But now he knew something had to change.

After several sessions of discussing what was happening at work, I asked Paul to tell me about his childhood. At first he talked about his father, a 1950s version of a deadbeat dad who seldom paid child support. In his home, to Paul and his brother and sister, being out of money and not knowing when or if the next check would arrive had come to seem normal.

He also talked about his mother, who was a well-loved figure in their small community—the kindly preschool teacher who listened to everybody's problems and seldom asked for anything for herself. Saint Margaret, his family and friends called her. Paul recalled his mother's struggle as a single parent who could never quite pay all the bills. Perhaps the most poignant and telling memory, however, was of the annual Christmas pageant at his mother's school, and a song the children sang each year. The words went like this: "If you want to be happy on Christmas Day, give something away, give something away. If you want to be happy on Christmas Day, give something you love away."

As we talked, the script came clear. In order to feel congruent with the world he had experienced as a child, Paul had to give it all away, not just at Christmas, but all the time. He also had to keep himself in a state of perpetual exhaustion and uncertainty, never quite sure if he could get it all done or meet all the financial obligations he'd taken on. No wonder Paul was dragging himself around in a late Stage 4 after being in his new job for less than two years.

In order to break that pattern, Paul had to work hard in several areas. First, he had to commit to some very different budgeting and spending habits. Next he enlisted the help of his wife and two friends to remind him to say no more often and pace himself. Finally, he met with his boss to map out a more limited but better-targeted marketing plan for the next quarter. At first he worried that he wouldn't have any friends left if he wasn't always available and couldn't afford lavish entertaining and gifts. And he wondered if he could do the job satisfactorily without being in overdrive all the time. But amazingly, nobody defected, and he didn't fail at work. He did, however, soon feel a lot more in control of his own life. What's more, his recurrent bronchitis cleared up. He was back in a Stage 2 place, determined to stay alert to the signals from his body and the people in his life.

And Rusting Out?

It's about a search ... for daily meaning as well as daily
bread, for recognition as well as cash, for astonishment
rather than torpor; in short, for a life rather than a Monday
through Friday sort of dying. —STUDS TERKEL

Rustout is a simpler problem, with less psychological unraveling
required. It's caused by staying in one place too long, without
enough challenge and intellectual lubrication. You must remember
that a "career" actually has three quite distinct parts: not only (1)
your current job or jobs, but also (2) ongoing education and training, and (3) networking in your current or related fields. Anything
you do to shake things up in any *one* of those areas has the capability of creating new energy in your career generally. Particularly
in these economic times, when job searches have become so prolonged, it's great to know that new learning or a targeted networking
effort can often spell relief while you keep on looking.

For instance, when Polly talked about how bored she was with
her work as a university administrator, she assumed that she'd have
to leave the university and the security she had established there to
find a job with a steeper learning curve. She was also upset at having had the flu three times in one season, and suspected that her
lack of interest in her work was wearing her down. But she was
conflicted. She had a daughter about to go to college, and the tuition assistance plan was attractive. Still, she felt that if she stayed
in her current position another four years without a break or some
new inspiration, she'd go nuts.

Polly was relieved to learn about career revitalization—which
certainly fit into her general life plan better than a major move. It
was fairly simple to devise an educational jump-start for her. She
would take advantage of the courses available right under her nose,
starting by auditing an art history course the next semester. She
would also sign up for advanced computer training workshops that
would help her with some of the database-management projects she
was working on. At first she worried that her boss wouldn't be able
to see any relationship between art history and her job. But he was

smart enough to know that the intellectual stimulation of the course would carry over to Polly's work and increase her connection to students and the college.

The plan turned out to be a good blend of the practical and the inspirational. In addition to helping with her daughter's tuition, it gave her some time to decide what next steps she might like to take. She also decided to do some networking by joining an area-wide women administrators' breakfast group. There Polly found other women wrestling with similar issues in their jobs. She enjoyed meeting with them once a month as a group and having lunches with individuals from the group now and again. Talking about different approaches to the same problems on different campuses brought new energy to her work. Suddenly she wasn't so eager to leave. As expected, it was back to Stage 2 for Polly.

Stage 4 Alert—Micromending

Organizations that stifle leadership from employees are no longer winning. —John Kotter

Individual workers are not the only people who have something at stake in the career-revitalization curve. Managers need to be concerned also. It's costly enough for organizations to lose once-competent individuals, in whom many training dollars have already been invested, and to hire and train someone new. But sometimes entire teams can sink into a numbing Stage 4 malaise, with devastating consequences for the health and effectiveness of the group.

Terms like *reengineering* and *work redesign* appear constantly in the pages of magazine articles and management books. Increasingly, companies are making it their business to develop programs for serving both the worker and the bottom line. But most of the award-winning programs touted by the media require large, system-wide changes. In board meetings all across the nation, many are discussed, but few are ever chosen for implementation. The inescapable fact is this: most of you will be working someplace else or will be retired before your organization is retooled in a way that really addresses employee needs. For that reason, the strategies I'm suggesting are *micro* rather than *macro*, small changes and fine-tunings that you can suggest now in your immediate work unit. Each of them has proven its ability to bring relief to the pain many of you might be feeling about your work. This might be a good time for you and your boss to have a "positive conspiracy" conversation about changing the Stage 4 state of mind in your unit, by introducing one or more of the following seven career-revitalization strategies.

Staying Alive at Work:
Seven Ways to Revitalize Your Career

You can sometimes fool the fans, but you can never fool the players. —Jack Stack

Swap Shops

We've already observed that a steep learning curve is good for your health and your productivity. What better way is there to keep learning than to take on different tasks periodically? For a decade now, industry has been proving that "universal operators" give work units the flexibility they need to respond to seasonal or unexpected demands. Workers who are trained to do different tasks, or whose job descriptions change in response to new challenges for their work unit, stay more engaged than their locked-in counterparts, provided that they are informed of impending changes and given the training they need to do their jobs well. I've talked to sales people, systems analysts, teachers, office workers, consumer product developers, nurses, and construction supervisors, to name a few, who have gotten out of Stage 4 by swapping parts of their regular jobs with others, so I know it works. If you're a little tired of doing your job the same old way, why not ask around in your unit about what new tasks might interest people and see what potential variations in how jobs are configured turn up?

In my experience, the best designers (and redesigners) of jobs are always the people doing the work. As Robert Waterman, author of *What America Does Right: Learning from Companies That Put People First,* observes, top-performing companies are committed to meeting the needs of their people, organizing downward rather than upward.[1] Here's that same old theme: the responsibility for letting your boss know what you need is clearly yours. Tell your boss that varying assignments to keep interest and learning high is one of many ways to keep you and your colleagues healthy and productive, while meeting the organization's need for productivity or profitability. As CEO Robert Ferchat suggests, "Free people to innovate so that your company can grow. Creativity is not the divine right of management."[2]

Teaming

Another worker-friendly strategy is teaming. You could be experiencing bursts of energy and creativity by converting some individual tasks to team efforts. On the surface, deploying several people in the place of one may seem inefficient, but people who divide up their jobs are then freed up for other projects. They are also energized, not only for that job but for others.

Teams, of course, have to learn team skills and practice them. They have to listen to each other to keep communication about what is expected of each person clear at all times. Teams are also fertile ground for organizations learning to do "systems thinking," unraveling the twisted knots of a messy problem back to their core sources. Different perspectives, shared in an atmosphere of mutual respect, will always get a better result than Lone Ranger approaches. According to *Fortune* magazine, more than half of America's large corporations are experimenting with self-managed teams. That's a productivity trend that you and your organization would do well to learn to ride.

New Digs

All of you have experienced the invigoration of rearranging your home or moving to a new one. So why not liven up your current office or even trade off work spaces with colleagues from time to time? The status quo in these little things can result in suffocating sameness without your even noticing it—and yet how easy it is, really, to arrange for a little fresh air. The renewal can be as simple as a few new plants and shoving some chairs and file cabinets around. Other times, entire units have been reconfigured and relocated. Whether the changes are large or small, it's the simple act of paying attention to your physical surroundings and doing something about them that brings a dose of personal power and revitalization. When your work slides over into Stage 4 toxicity, you forget the little things that can make big differences. I've seen whole work teams transformed by such renovations.

Flexibility

Workers have quite different demands on their time, with obligations not only to their job but to their children, relationships, aging parents, continuing education, and community, to name a few of the possibilities. How can employees and their managers collaborate to soften the inevitable collisions between work and those other roles? One way is staggered starts and finishes to the workday, or schedule variations such as working four long days rather than five regular ones, either periodically or consistently. But when you're dragging around in late Stage 4, it's hard to remember to propose such innovations.

Telecommuting is another growing alternative. Charles Rodgers of Work/Family Directions, a Boston consulting firm that helps corporations develop more family-friendly strategies, estimates that more than 20 percent of jobs could easily be done from home. Increasingly, even corporate giants are turning to telecommuting as a way to reduce overhead. One telecommuting financial analyst keeps all the company documents she'll need to do her work at home in a looseleaf notebook labeled "Virtual Home Office."

Flexibility can be a delicate issue, particularly in a work unit with an inflexible boss. In these situations, workers often compete with each other for tiny shreds of approval and rewards. Each worker waits petulantly for a sign that others are getting more than their fair share. Flexibility, perceived as "special treatment" in that shutdown context, can cause many problems. On the other hand, when the supervisor makes it clear that all requests for individual flexibility will be evaluated in terms of their ability to enhance both individual and group effectiveness, then much more is possible. Work/Family Directions has in fact created a form for workers in their organization to use in requesting more flexible arrangements—requiring them to demonstrate the positive impact of the desired change on their own and the office's productivity. In this context, workers are free to suggest variations that could be energizing for everyone, and fewer people sit around collecting evidence that things aren't fair.

Some people get nervous when you talk about individual flexibility. They usually argue that consistency is the only way to ensure equality of treatment and fairness for all. Well, treating people with different needs in a compulsively uniform manner, thereby *ignoring* their needs, is actually the least "fair" thing managers can do. And it diminishes the employees' desire to go the extra mile when supervisors need them to.

One fail-safe way to oversee the fairness with which supervisors administer the flexibility in their work units is to allow for safe bottom-up feedback to managers. This can be done through anonymous individual written evaluations, submitted to the supervisor and then on up the chain of command. At Federal Express, for instance, top managers receive (or don't receive) hefty annual bonuses based on the responses to employee surveys about whether they feel they have been treated with respect by their supervisors. Since compensation for these leaders often includes bonuses of up to 40 percent of their base salary, you can bet they pay close attention to the needs of their employees.

According to the director of research at Catalyst, a New York City–based research and advocacy firm for women in business, "the resistance of middle managers continues to be the single biggest obstacle to the use of flexible work arrangements."[3] In 1989, few organizations offered flexible schedules, but four years later, a study found that 38 percent of companies interviewed by Catalyst had more than a hundred employees in a flexible mode. In those organizations, human resource specialists had warned that choosing to work flexible schedules would have dire consequences for employees' careers. In reality, just the opposite happened: more than half of the workers interviewed got promoted after changing to flexible hours.

Initiating Novices

A real win-win situation for both individuals and teams is inviting interns and apprentices into your organization. Interns provide a tremendous amount of free or inexpensive labor. They free up regular employees to do new tasks, and enable work units to complete "wish list" tasks that otherwise wouldn't get done, such as completing research projects, writing manuals or other publications, and planning for special events or other department initiatives. But there are positive effects for individual workers as well. Teaching eager novices what you know about your field gives you a chance to mentor others and feel good about yourself in the process. Your body reacts positively to reaching out to others, as well as to the self-appreciation that being a mentor brings. Training and mentoring others also improves your skills by calling attention to your own performance; you grow because you concentrate more on your work, rather than performing job functions in an automatic way. What's more, interns bring organizations fresh perspectives and questions about why you do things certain ways. Given the learning/relearning requirements for staying current in this runaway economic environment, some good questions from a bright outsider are probably one of the best things that could happen to your work unit.

Strategic Support Groups

These informally constituted groups (maximum number in a group is ten) are much neglected tools for taking care of yourself, for knowing when you're falling into a Stage 4 mindset, and for growing in your career. They are priceless forums for discussing new ideas, solving problems, and sharing feedback. If you haven't been in one, you have been missing a terrific opportunity. Honest, insightful feedback about how you're doing in your job and how you're perceived may be the best gift anybody can give you. Strategic support groups are an invaluable form of peer coaching, but they are not to be taken lightly. You should form or join one only if you're willing to make a commitment of loyalty and confidentiality to each member. These few basic rules can make your group maximally helpful:

- Meet regularly at a mutually acceptable time and place. Protect that time jealously!
- Keep a three-to-one ratio of strategizing to complaining. (A little kvetching goes a long way.) You might want to practice some of Seligman's ABCDE disputation from Chapter 4 if anybody seems to be turning the negativity on herself or himself.
- If you're in the same organization, support each other's achievements or points of view whenever appropriate in meetings, conferences, or informal conversations. Send congratulatory memos with copies to the "right" people when one of your group does something important for the organization.
- Commit to giving feedback and other relevant information to your support group associates within twenty-four hours of hearing about it. This one is tough to do, but it is essential.
- Have homework—readings to discuss and follow-up tasks for each member to complete and report back on at the next session. This one is particularly important if one of your goals is helping one or more people in the group make a career change.

Four female middle managers in a consumer products firm arrived in my office one day, saying they wanted to convert their group from a support group, "where all we do is moan," to a more problem-solving mode. The strategic support group ground rules were all they needed to get started. The three-to-one guideline got them on track right away. They checked back in periodically to let me know that they had enlarged the group to seven, and that all seven of them were feeling less stressed because they had begun to see real results on the job.

"Remembering to spread good news about each other has been the most important change for me," one group member said. "Not for me," said another. "It was that feedback rule—what a difference it's made in helping me to face and learn from my mistakes."

More Supervision

"What, are you crazy?" a work group once asked when I suggested they ask their boss for more specific coaching and supervision. The fact is, though, that when managers are actively coaching you, sharing what they know, and encouraging you to set performance goals and sharpen your skills, it's very invigorating. There are several processes involved in good coaching—which is very different from the toxic gatekeeping that many managers seem to be doing.

The first step is for managers to establish a positive relationship with employees, based on a clear understanding of each one's strengths. This means a commitment to perceiving and valuing their particular abilities, even when some workers' styles are antithetical to the supervisor's. It also means understanding that the stylistic weaknesses workers bring to the job are usually excesses of their strengths. The enthusiastic, spontaneous idea-generator type worker will probably not be as organized and good at follow-through. On the other hand, the conscientious, organized, detail-oriented worker will very likely not turn ideas on their heads often enough to stay competitive. When they're both working collaboratively on the same team, however, both the *front end* and *back end* will be covered.

In the coaching process, after relationship-building comes shared goal-setting, to help you improve in the areas in which you're underdeveloped. The literature of motivation is very clear on this point: learners of all kinds need to believe in and develop goals themselves in order to excel.

The third step is pointing out examples for the worker to emulate. Sometimes they are the coach's own skills, sometimes those of other people. Additional training is also usually indicated—a workshop in time management, a creativity seminar, a writing course, or a series of computer trainings, for instance.

The final step to the process, then, is follow-through. You make progress on the goals, and your supervisor stays involved to monitor and reward your progress. As a result, you back out of Stage 4, and your unit benefits.

Music, Maestro!

Most of us try to sing the note we like best or the note we've been told to sing, but the sound is usually muffled because it's not our note.   —PETER ELBOW

"Revitalized work" charges you with staying alive and alert to what songs you want to be singing in your career. It requires you to become responsible for managing your own work space and work relationships, to fit not only the goals of the office but also what matters and feels right to you. Most people know how they like their coffee in the morning, but surprisingly few have taken the time to consider what office environment, or schedule, or kinds of interactions at work might be the most naturally energizing for them. Have you?

In most organizations, that kind of introspection and analysis has seldom been encouraged, particularly at a time when the prevailing assumption is "Just be glad you *have* a job." But when you don't know what you need, you can't try to make it happen. Instead, you stay in passive modes of "Fix it for me" or "Don't bother, it's hopeless," and wonder why work gets sickening.

Every one of the health-care professionals I have interviewed over the past several years has told me of their offices being crammed with patients whose bodies are in pain because they are tired of their jobs, and yearning for some flexibility and new challenges to get them energized about their work again. Indeed, unless workers and managers figure out how to put aside their differences and become co-conspirators in a campaign to keep work revitalized, we're all in for a lot more emotional and physical suffering.

6. Does Your Work Still Fit?

Nothing in the world can make up for the lack of joy in one's work. —SIMONE WEIL

If you didn't find yourself in the chapter on stuck people and you've tried different things to revitalize your career, yet you still have a haunting feeling you're in the wrong job—well, perhaps you are! It's really not very difficult to end up in a job that doesn't fit. Sometimes you just outgrow what you've been doing. Few people would try to wear most of the clothes they bought decades ago. People's tastes and dimensions often change over time. And yet many of you are probably making yourselves unhappy and unhealthy by squeezing yourselves into career decisions made long ago.

Others of you are probably in situations that don't fit because someone else chose it for you or your work has changed around you. You'd have to search hard to find an organization that hasn't been buffeted by some sort of critical change—in people, structure, or products—in the past several years. Staffing turnovers always upend your work world, particularly when a new supervisor or co-worker whose style doesn't fit with yours enters the scene. Every organization is also asking much more of its workers, in terms of work to be done and levels of skills to be mastered. Some people love new challenges, while others resist changing old patterns, as we discussed in Chapter 4. For any of these reasons, therefore, you may be caught in an ill-fitting work situation that is becoming toxic for you.

An old proverb says, "If you choose a job you love, you'll never work a day in your life." In the past several decades I've watched many people achieve this, even after they had given up on ever finding work that could make them happy. Perhaps you believe that if any parts of your work still fit, you'll just have to put up with the parts that don't, particularly now, when friends and family members are reminding you how lucky you are even to have a job. But trying to ignore the parts of a job that don't work well for you now can only make you miserable and ill eventually. Here's a checklist to help you get some idea how poor the fit really is for you now.

Do You Really Have to Go Now?

Put a check next to any of the "symptoms" below which are currently true for you.

_____ Strong feelings of betrayal by your employer or by an individual at work

_____ Difficulty sleeping

_____ Anger you can't seem to shake

_____ A negative relationship with your supervisor

_____ Withdrawal of support from your organization—i.e., loss of resources, diminished assignments

_____ Negative feedback about your performance

_____ Recurrent physical problems

_____ Frequent feelings of impatience and irritability

_____ Boredom

_____ Impaired personal life due to excessive work demands

_____ Increased eating, spending, smoking, alcohol intake, use of prescription drugs in response to work pressures

_____ Unpleasant relationships with co-workers

_____ Consistent feelings of incompetence or irrelevance

____ Lack of joy about your work

____ Persistent feelings of being undervalued

____ Recurrent depression, sadness

____ Lack of meaning in your work

____ Persistent fatigue

____ Feeling that your work is out of control

____ Feeling dead-ended at work

____ Anxiety, fearfulness

____ Being passed over for important assignments or promotion

____ Frustration with how things are run

____ Lack of time to do the things that matter to you

If you checked off four or fewer items, you're probably experiencing uncertainty like everyone else, but you seem to have your problems in hand. You might circle or write down the suggestions in the book that seem likely to work for you, and begin on at least one of them. It would be useful also to share your responses to this exercise with someone else, who agrees to check in with you about your progress.

If you checked between five and nine items, you're in the middle zone. Stress is high, but in all likelihood, enough things are going well to keep you afloat for now. It will be important, however, to pay careful attention to the VITAL formula in Chapter 7. And for you too, a buddy to check your progress is a good idea.

If you checked ten or more, this is a May Day alert. It's time to make major changes or prepare to leave. You should be taking notes in all the margins of this book.

Call It Failing or Call It Learning?

Our life is the path of learning to wake up before we die.
—NATALIE GOLDBERG

Maybe your job doesn't fit because you didn't get enough information before making the decision to take it. You really can't know if you're going to like artichokes until you taste them. The same is true of jobs many times; you need a chance to experience them firsthand.

David was one of the people who hadn't found out enough about what his new position as director of technical support in a small financial services firm would really be like, because the job was offered to him when his supervisor left and he was too shocked and flattered to ask many questions. It seemed clear to him that refusing the position would alienate his boss, the chief information officer, and besides, he really needed the money. A year later, it felt like half the world was watching when he finally got up the nerve to inform his boss that his skyrocketing blood pressure and sleepless nights were telling him that this new position just didn't work for him. Before his physical discomfort forced him to face the truth and do something about it, however, David spent several months obsessively reviewing every "failure" he could dig out of his memory bank. He even remembered the gruesome details of the spelling bee he lost in front of the entire seventh grade. As you can imagine, when he finally got to my office, his self-esteem was badly tattered. The questions David and I used to find out what was wrong for him at work might be helpful to you as well. You can apply the following *questions of fit* to either the job you have now or one you left and would like to understand better.

Questions of Fit

I don't believe you live the good life by doing what you *can* do; you live it by doing what you *want* to do.
—Barbara Sher

The questions in this section require quiet time alone, as well as some in-depth discussions with people who know you well. It would also be useful for you to write out the answers, date them, and file them for future reference in your career log. Career mismatches usually take a long time to acknowledge and an even longer time to put behind you. But they have tremendous potential for learning and growth. Hopefully, you're getting the message by now that the career log process is an important, ongoing tool for staying in control of your own career. So are these questions of fit: you should plan on thinking about them early and often throughout your career.

1. In what ways is the job a good fit for you?
2. What are you asked to do in the job that doesn't really fit you?
3. What skills and interests of yours don't fit in your job?
4. What values of yours don't fit with the obligations of that position?
5. What about you seems very different from others in your work group?
6. How do the demands of this position fit with the rest of your life? What is the cost to your emotional and physical health?
7. What are you looking for that you haven't gotten?
8. What was your hidden fantasy going into this position? Will you seek it again in your next job, or is it time to give up the fantasy?

Once David got over being ashamed and feeling he had disappointed his boss, he was ready to act on the answers he had given to the questions I had posed. In some ways the job *had* been a good fit, since he was clearly the best technical problem-solver in the organization. His boss had therefore concluded that he should head up the technical team. But the job was also a supremely poor fit because David didn't want to be a boss. He was very bright, introverted, and loyal; he took his relationships seriously and didn't want to have to give negative feedback to people he really liked. He also loved to go off on tangents with interesting technical problems; in fact, he cared much more about the intricacies of the technology than about the profitability of the company. At unit head meetings, he had frequently felt as if he lived in a world far removed from the other directors.

David finally figured out that he had been seduced by the confidence his boss seemed to have in him. He had kept hidden even from himself the memories of his father leaving home when he was in first grade, and the seemingly endless hours he spent after that waiting for him to come to visit and see how well he was doing in school. Being the technical whiz kid in his firm now finally gave him the fatherly approval for which he had longed. But this position also required him to manage rather than be the creative technical thinker—in fact, his constant supply of new ideas often got in the way when a major project needed to be nailed down. When that happened, and he was on the receiving end of needling memos or comments, he would often despair and wonder whether he was really very good at anything.

As we talked about his options, David concluded that he didn't want to leave his company. He had friends there and he saw many interesting technical problems still to be solved. And so he gathered his courage and asked his boss if he could have a different kind of position, as an internal consultant of sorts, where he would be free to roam as a problem-solver and occasional project manager, rather than the permanent team leader and supervisor. During that terrifying but exciting session, he laid out many ideas he'd like to explore that he thought might increase the efficiency and effectiveness of their systems.

David's boss was taken back and disappointed at first, but he didn't want to lose David—he found many of his new suggestions quite fascinating! Even though resources were tight, he told David he'd try to find a way to divide up the director's job to give him the kind of position he wanted. Within the month David had a newly created position as senior technical adviser that fit him much better—and the technical group had a manager who wanted to manage.

David's situation raises the interesting question of which concerns should matter most to an organization—yours or the organization's? Could employers realize their goals better by paying closer attention to what employees need? Performance management and motivation research shouts loud and clear: "Yes!" When employees believe that the organization is responding to what will "fit" them best, they reward the organization through more commitment, more work, and more creativity. Trying to get that notion understood by both employees and their supervisors, however, is often a hard sell. Fortunately, David's boss was able to grasp the concept, and he did both the company and David a big favor by tailoring the job to the extraordinary skills of his young computer whiz.

What Makes For a Bad Fit?

Zen is the game of insight, the game of discovering who you are beneath the social masks. —REGINALD BLYTH

The possibilities for good and bad fits are infinite, and the question is made even more perplexing because fit is so often a developmental issue—you just keep on changing, whether you want to or not. Sometimes the way you're changing fits well with the direction in which the organization or work unit is moving. That's a real win-win when it happens. But sometimes the combinations are not so positive.

Among the countless ways in which your evolving needs and the demands of your work can conflict, four kinds of mismatches are common:

- Neglected aptitudes
- Not enough fun
- Not enough safety and affirmation
- Wrong rhythm

Neglected Aptitudes

Aptitudes: When they aren't used, they begin to itch, making you bored, dissatisfied, and restless. Aptitudes are both a blessing and a curse. It feels great to hone a skill you already have, or to uncover and nurture a talent or interest from long ago. With good supports, many people rediscover talents they deserted in their younger years. But when aptitudes are not used, they begin to itch, making you bored, dissatisfied, and restless.

This is particularly true for aptitudes that are less "practical" in nature—the singing voice or poetry writing or public speaking or athletic ability you turned your back on in favor of ways to make a more secure living, for instance. When I ask, "What did you used to love to do in school or college that you haven't done in years?" people almost always offer a heartfelt reply:

- "Designing the sets for our class plays, but I haven't picked up a paint brush since senior year."
- "I was a natural athlete as a kid. I remember the trophies for soccer and tennis in my bedroom, but there's not time for that in my life now."
- "I was great at math, but because I was a girl, I was discouraged from taking advanced courses. I've always wondered what I missed."

Sometimes such talents can indeed be developed and integrated into a career; at other times they are more appropriate for extra-career activities. Wherever you decide to put them, however, they need to be noticed. Ignoring them just won't work. The low-level stress that comes from selling out your own talents will culminate in some form of physical discomfort.

Milton was clearly a case in point. He came to my office through an outplacement referral, after he was laid off from his job as an accountant. He arrived talking about how exhausted he felt, his aches and pains punctuated by herpes outbreaks.

Milton had become an accountant because he was really good at math and his parents had said that it would be a logical choice. In college he had gotten a bachelor's degree in business, with a concentration in finance and accounting. When an accounting firm came to his college and offered him a job, it seemed like the appropriate thing to do to take it. He stayed with that same company for nearly twenty years, until he was laid off in a sweep of downsizing. He reported feeling surprised that his reaction to his pink slip had been more relief than anger.

I asked Milton what other courses besides the numbers-oriented ones he had enjoyed in college. I was not surprised when he paused to take in the question—Milton was nothing if not measured and serious about everything. But I was shocked when he broke out in a grin. "I've always loved words," he said, "but my family and teachers convinced me that I was a numbers person, mostly because there was something practical you could do with numbers. Every once in a while, I sit down and write a letter to the editor or to some public official, and it feels pretty good." He continued, "Then I wonder about being a writer. But immediately my common sense tells me what a stupid idea that is. How could I trade in my salary and security for a life as an impoverished writer?"

At that point Milton and I talked about what I call my *collage theory of career design*. I explained that we are used to taking *photographs* of our work lives—clear, crisp pictures of a particular job, as in doctor, lawyer, banker—a title that defines (and delimits) our daily activities. Only our titles and job descriptions fit into the frame. When we do that, we often cut out of the frame those things (such as an interest in writing) that don't fit the dominant paradigm.

On the canvas of a *collage*, however, there are several, or even many, splashes of color—some in the center, some off-center, some large, some small. Some are brightly colored, while others are more subtle. This is a total picture of the things you love to do. Some are part of your paid work, and others are not. Throughout your career, when you allow them to, the shape, size, and intensity of your splashes of color change as they rearrange themselves in your life. Your job is to keep checking your canvas, to see what's wanting to happen there. For years Milton's work as an accountant had been the dominant figure on his canvas, its size and density blocking out almost everything else.

Milton's writing, however, could easily have become part of his work with his firm, had he taken it seriously, availed himself of some further training, and then proposed that he do some writing of reports as part of his job. Had he been more forthcoming about wanting to develop more of his talents, perhaps he might have been seen differently by his employer. Ironically, one of the reasons Milton got his pink slip was because he was perceived to be one-dimensional, excessively obedient, and not likely to want to try new things.

Once he awoke to the possibilities inherent in his new freedom, he discovered several hidden colors to add to his collage. In addition to the writing, he found that he really liked young people. He enjoyed teaching Sunday school, and talked about maybe adding some kind of teaching to his collage. Ever so gradually Milton had to admit that this whole thing was turning out all right. He was having more fun thinking about his work than he had in a very long time.

Of course, the American proclivity for spending often makes it hard for people to take the time for reflection and planning, as well as the time for the retraining needed to enliven their collage. Fortunately, Milton's accountant discipline had protected him on this score, and so he and his wife, Peg, had enough put away to get them through a period of re-evaluation.

The collage that Milton proudly displayed eighteen months after his dismissal was surely different from the picture I saw when we first met. He had taken three semesters of writing instruction with a local writing teacher and had a portfolio with a wide range of writing samples. He had also been volunteering at a nearby independent school as a math tutor and having a great deal of success; he had just agreed to be the adviser for a business careers club the next semester.

Perhaps the biggest surprise of all, however, was how much Milton enjoyed having more time at home with his three teenagers. Peg, meanwhile, had decided to get her MBA at night, leaving a large hole in the family's domestic management plan. Milton stepped in. The boys learned about cooking and cleanup, and his daughter got some lessons in emergency appliance repair. The whole family came alive with the new arrangements.

Milton's story is always with me when I urge people to sock

away some money in case they need to invest in their own growth someday. Good recovery plans take time, and the longer you can give yourself, the better off you'll be. Milton's collage, by the way, came together with some very splashy designs. After investigating the range of desktop publishing packages available, he invested in some equipment and began learning how to do newsletters, brochures, and such. He also expanded his work at the school, and after two years of volunteering there, was hired as a part-time math teacher. Private schools often require people to wear several hats, so Milton was also able to contract for occasional work in the business office and the development office, using both his accounting and his writing skills. Of course he wasn't making as much money as he had as a more-than-full-time accountant, but Peg was about to make more with the completion of her business degree. Overall, the family financial picture wouldn't be much different than before. But the family itself was much different. And as you might expect, Milton had far fewer herpes outbreaks.

Like Milton, you might not have allowed yourself to think about your favorite talents and aptitudes in a long time. Promise yourself that sometime in the next week you'll make a list of your talents (maybe even during a brainwalking exercise), and check to see how many of them are currently on your career or life collage. Sooner or later, the neglected ones will haunt you.

Not Enough Fun

Fun: You need it at work more than ever! If you're not having fun at work, you're working at the wrong place, or you're working at the right place but in the wrong way. I'm always amazed at the incredible range of things that people consider fun. Whether fun for you means solving seemingly impossible problems or organizing messes or sharing your newest jokes with an appreciative audience, one thing is for certain: you've got to find ways to have some of it at work. Particularly when trying to survive the toxicity of the nineties.

The first thing to do is to really believe that work should be fun.

Some of us learned from family members who survived the Depression or whose own work has been mundane or monotonous that work is a form of duty rather than something to be enjoyed. Once that erroneous assumption has been set aside, however, there are lots of things you can do to bring lightness and humor to work with you. Finding some soulmates will be critical if you're fun-deprived. Go to other departments or work teams if your own is full of stuffed shirts, but by all means find people to have lunch with, take walks with, exchange interesting and humorous e-mail with, and generally lighten things up a little. Corporations and nonprofits all around the country have figured out that humor helps people to work more effectively and keeps them healthier. Humor consultants are doing a brisk business everywhere. If your organization hasn't gotten that message yet, you might want to consult some of the many resources in bookstores to share with your boss or your human resources department, whoever seems more likely to listen.

A good way to check for pleasure at work is, as creativity consultants teach work teams to do, to ask a big *what if?* question. Ask yourself this: *What if my salary were determined by how much pleasure I get from my work?* Then take the exercise a step further, and generate some answers to this question: *If I could earn the most money by having the most fun, what activities/tasks/functions would I be pushing to schedule into my workday?* Then add the next question: *And how much would I be earning* now? The answers you get will tell you a lot about what's missing in your work.

Not Enough Safety and Affirmation

Affirmation: Feeling that you belong at work is critical. It's said about family life that being born is like being invited to a party and arriving when the activities are already in full swing: you spend the rest of your life figuring out what's going on and how to fit in successfully. Well, the same metaphor applies to the "families" at work. Sometimes you find out that the "style" of the party fits you very well; and at other times you might find yourself marginalized or left out. You may also have fit in once, but find now that the rules and some of the players have changed, leaving you much less comfortable than before. Or as we pointed out earlier, you might find that you have been the one doing the changing. It doesn't matter whether you changed or the place changed. If the prevailing environment of your work unit is not one which makes you feel appreciated and able to trust the people around you, then it's time to look elsewhere.

Below are some statements to help you assess how much affirmation and sense of belonging you feel you are getting from the "family" at work. How true is each of these statements for you?

- My boss lets me know that my work and my style are appreciated.
- I know that my co-workers respect me.
- I am able to relax and be myself at work.
- I feel comfortable sharing details of my personal life at work.
- It's easy for me to laugh at work.
- I trust my boss.
- I trust my co-workers.
- It's easy for me to collaborate on projects with others at work.
- My boss's management style fits with how I prefer to work.
- I believe that my ideas are sought after and respected at work.

Note that the first two statements refer to *what you've been told about your value*. Some of you work in an organization in which you are indeed valued, but the style of the organization is not to tell people good things. I once asked the executive director of an organization where I was consulting on morale issues why he never told people how much he valued them. His response was that the lawyer they consulted for personnel crises had told them it was better to keep employees a little off-balance and to keep praise minimal in case they needed to lay people off eventually. In that way, there would probably be less trouble with grievances, he had advised. In reality, most of the employees there actually were quite competent, but nobody had bothered to tell them. No wonder they were now paying consultants to figure out how to fix the environment which that mind-set had created. So if the first two statements are not true for you, you might want to check into whether it's a problem of valuing or a problem with giving appropriate feedback.

One possibility to be considered is that you are getting validation but not taking it in. There are analogies in biology. With one form of diabetes, for instance, the body doesn't make enough insulin to meet our needs. In another form, however, the body produces enough but doesn't use it effectively. So too with positive reinforcement. If it's there but you're not using it well, some sessions with a counselor about why it's hard for you to believe good things about yourself or hold on to positive feelings for very long are probably in order.

The other statements are all related to how easy it feels to be in your work family. Think back to the days of early family life: we like to think our families were magical, but actually most of them ended up shortchanging us to some degree in one way or another. Some of you might have lived in family units where one or two of the members ended up as scapegoats for the whole unit—by focusing attention on how they didn't fit in, it was possible to ignore problems with the system as a whole. The same thing happens in work units. If you're in a situation where you're being scapegoated, or where your style really doesn't fit the prevailing fashion of how people ought to be, then your self-esteem must be in trouble (or soon will be) and it's not healthy for you to stay there much longer.

If you work in a place where there's not much appreciation coming your way, for one reason or another, there are some practical manipulations to try before you abandon ship. One suggestion is to have a talk with your supervisor about his perceptions of your work and your concern about not being valued. I've seen new levels of awareness and cooperation on both sides spring from those kinds of candid discussions.

Another approach is to make a careful assessment of the people who seem to be the most like you—the ones who seem to do their work the same way as you and value or enjoy the same things. Whether they're in your immediate work unit or elsewhere in the organization, find a way to talk to them, invite them to lunch, or sit together at events or meetings. Don't just hope you'll run into them: make a *strategic plan* for getting enough contact with people like yourself. Being for even a little while in the company of people wired the same way you are can make a tremendous difference in how it feels to go to work. When your job has become too tight and toxic for you, it's easy to forget to be proactive.

If you can find professional or business organizations to join, you'll have a chance to learn new things, meet new people, and line up a few like-minded colleagues. This is something you should be doing anyway, whether work feels undermining or not, because constant exposure to different ways of doing things is essential to staying vital. But it's critically important for you if your primary workplace is a depleter rather than a recharger for you. This strategy has the added benefit of helping you get ready to escape the emptiness and find a new job.

Another reason that some employees find it hard to feel safe and affirmed is the pervasive discrimination which manages to hang on in organizations. Even in these rapidly changing times, the majority of tradition-bound organizations still clone themselves when it comes to hiring and promoting people. Even though it's illegal to do so, the desire to choose and reward people who make the people in charge feel comfortable is almost irresistible. This leaves those who don't fit the dominant norms feeling like second-class citizens. Moreover, when things get tight in organizations and people turn on each other, the soil is fertile for discrimination.

In many organizations, women are still battling for the right to be rewarded equally, despite the fact that more women than men go to college, and research shows that women are better students and more productive employees than men.[1] Research from the American Association of University Women has shown over and over, for instance, that girls don't get a fair deal in mixed-gender educational settings, from preschool all the way through graduate and professional school. My own firsthand observations have certainly borne that out. In consultations with surgical residents who were completing their training, I was informed by bitter young women that they were regularly embarrassed by older surgeons on the hospital staff and criticized much more than their fellow male residents. One very competent young female surgeon reported that she had been admonished to "never again tie a knot like a girl."

Treating females like second-class citizens doesn't end with the classroom or training program. In interviews with CEOs for Fortune 1,000 companies, 80 percent of the men interviewed admitted that gender discrimination in their organizations kept women from realizing their full potential. Those CEOs with any program or process in place at the time to deal with the problem, however, were fewer than 1 percent.[2] Women in for-profit and nonprofit organizations alike feel like outsiders and find it hard to sustain their commitment because of compromised opportunities at work. One particularly unfortunate outcome of the backlash women are experiencing seems to come from a pairing of resentment against what is sometimes perceived as reverse discrimination with fears of sexual-harassment allegations. Mentoring is a critical component of career success; neither men nor women can climb the career ladder without it. In the current environment, however, men are reluctant to appear to be making even professional overtures to women, for fear of being misunderstood. As one male executive admitted, increasingly fewer men are willing to risk inviting women behind closed doors in their offices for the kind of honest feedback you need for effective mentoring. That lack of coaching and support is making it even harder for achievement-oriented women to feel truly engaged with their organizations.

You may have noticed—the politics of the mid-nineties are often not friendly to non-mainstream people. And there are so many ways to be outside the parameters of the mainstream: not just gender, but race, ethnicity, religion, age, social class, sexual orientation, disabilities, and even appearance and personal style. Marianne, for instance, was a very successful director of corporate communications for a major bank in Chicago when we first met. She was smart, energetic, very attractive, and turning forty. She was also a very closeted lesbian. She had poignant stories to tell of trumped-up boyfriends, a closet full of sequined gowns she'd never dream of putting on in front of her friends, and innumerable required client parties to which she went alone, leaving her partner Jan at home. The VP to whom she reported thought she was terrific, as indeed she was, but Marianne knew that he had strong religious convictions about homosexuality, because he had mentioned them on several occasions. So she had concluded that there was no way she could be "out" at work. For the first five years she worked at the bank, that hadn't really mattered to her. She was still learning the business and it was good fodder for comedy routines with her friends to joke about the fake dates and sequins. But gradually that got old, and she began to resent the required evening events without Jan. She also began to hate the fact that it felt dishonest to her.

Some of her friends in other corporations had already taken a leap and told their colleagues and bosses about their gay lifestyle, with varying degrees of success. In some cases the boss was accepting and the air seemed clearer. In other situations, however, friends had found themselves mysteriously relegated to less important projects and not invited to important events. Marianne wasn't willing to take the chance that could lead to second-class citizenship at the bank. But she also wasn't willing to deny her personal life any longer. The paralysis she felt as a result of those conflicting motivations was what had brought her to me.

And so she marshaled all of the strategic planning and marketing skills that made her so good at her job into plotting her escape into a life where she could be herself. She explored other corporations with a reputation for welcoming diversity and had a round of interviews that seemed promising at first. But she finally decided that she'd get more of what she really wanted by opening her own communications firm and offering her services to a mix of mainstream and alternative organizations. She and Jan had to adjust their standard of living to plan for the new business, but that turned out to be easier than expected. Much to their surprise, they discovered that much of their prior spending had been in the service of *compensating* for the secrecy and dishonesty they were caught in, rather than for things they really needed.

Within a year her freelance business was launched part-time, and within one more year she was able to cut loose from the bank altogether. Little did the homophobic VP know that the posters and brochures he had liked so much now bore the same imprint as those for the Gay and Lesbian Alliance, the Peace Resources Group, and other organizations that Marianne had always wanted to support. I think of Marianne's signature logo on that startling array of brochures when anyone wonders aloud if it's really possible to leave an organization when the norms don't fit, to find a situation where you can really be engaged.

The story is not much different with people of color, people with disabilities, or people from working class or different ethnic backgrounds. Being different is not really safe, despite the legal protection afforded by nondiscrimination clauses. Going to court to win a discrimination case usually takes five to fifteen years of a person's life and often leaves a shattered professional reputation in its wake. Only the truly committed can withstand the ordeal.

Throughout life, remediation is harder than prevention. Therefore, the first piece of advice to people who feel outside the mainstream in some way is to choose carefully and look for employers where diversity and openness to different ideas are woven into the fabric of the organization. Lawrence Otis Graham spent two years compiling a list of eighty-five corporations that make a point to be welcoming to minority hires. In his book *The Best Companies for Minorities*, he identified organizations that are especially committed to finding, training, and promoting people of color. There are similar books written about corporate hospitality for women and for lesbians and gay men. This kind of "respect for difference" report card is critical to have, either formally or informally, in making career search decisions. There are other resources available to help job-seekers become knowledgeable about various organizations. *Business Ethics Magazine* is an excellent reporter on companies that understand the importance of respecting all workers. Business for Social Responsibility groups are also ready resources, as is the Conference Board's Diversity Council. If you attended a college or university with a strong alumni networking system, that's also a way to do some effective "insider" spying about acceptance of differences in various organizations.

The second suggestion for surviving in organizations where your status is "other" is to find a niche and be very good at what you do. Of course, it's unfair that people who are different have to strategize about their careers more than others. However, meeting these kinds of challenges develops your creativity and positions you well for the job market of the future. Those who spend time bemoaning the injustices rather than figuring out how to make them irrelevant are short-circuiting themselves, and probably compromising their health. People who are successful in any field today have used a kind of individualized strategic planning to analyze the following factors:

- What's needed, by a given employer or in the field generally
- What relevant skills they have to meet the need(s)
- How to position themselves to be tapped to fill the need(s)

If you sit outside the mainstream in your organization, the reality is that you'll probably need to be a bit more aggressive with this strategy. Remember, more than any other factor, being valued for what you bring to your organization will buy you permission to be different.

A final strategy is obvious. Find support; don't suffer in silence. It's important to have people who can understand what you're feeling, as well as commiserate and strategize with you. As one of my colleagues insists, "You gotta have a gang." Often it also helps your employer when you do. McDonald's won the 1993 Award of Excellence from Catalyst for their Women's Operators Network, an organization of female franchise owners who work together to share important information. They support each other in managing their franchises in a more employee-centered way. Profits from the female-managed restaurants have now outstripped those of the male-managed franchises. What's more, establishments run by women are so much safer that the women have been given permission to purchase their liability insurance separately from the men because they qualify for a lower rate.

Women in corporate headquarters at McDonald's are also organized. I spoke with a senior member of the Women's Leadership Network. She observed that while the network is newer than the women operators' group, members have already felt the desirable effects of feeling more connected to each other and to new strategic initiatives in play in the organization. Even though McDonald's is regarded as a progressive corporation and a good place for women to work, I was told, you can never have too much information or be too connected if you want to be steering your own career. So if something about you has you positioned outside the mainstream in your organization, don't give up, and don't go it alone. You're much less likely to find the engagement you and your employer need you to have on your own than in a group.

Wrong Rhythm

The body-mind effect of various factors is always modulated by the natural rhythms of the individual. Robert Ader, the scientist credited with first showing the interdependence of our immune and nervous systems, demonstrated how important it is for organisms to follow their own natural rhythms. In experiments testing the role of gastric-gland secretions in causing ulcers, Ader divided his rats into two groups: those who naturally secreted a great deal of the suspected ulcer-causing chemical pepsinogen and those who naturally secreted very little. Then he "stressed" both groups by restraining them. As expected, the rats who developed ulcers were primarily the ones who secreted the most pepsinogen. But not all of the rats who got ulcers were high-secreters. Ader discovered that rats have natural cycles of high and low activity, and that even low-secreters can develop ulcers when they are restrained during their own natural high-activity cycles. Thus, reasoned Ader and his associates, the body-mind effect of various factors is always modulated by the natural rhythms of the individual.[3] So if you're in a job that seems as if it ought to fit but you find yourself rattled at work more often than you'd like, pay some attention to the rhythm your body seems to want—when to be moving about, when to take it easy, and so forth. You may then need to have a talk with your supervisor about how to vary your routine—if you want to stay healthy, that is.

Much workplace distress can be attributed to rigid schedules and an overemphasis on conformity and consistency in the places where we work. I had a conversation with Marjorie Kelly, editor of *Business Ethics* magazine, on a hot summer morning. We were discussing the likelihood that organizations would ever be able to find ways to meet their short-term fiscal obligations and yet give their employees enough flexibility to work more in harmony with their own natural rhythms and abilities. Marjorie observed, "As I was hurrying and sweating my way to work this morning, I noticed that all the big, hairy dogs were going along at a snail's pace, stopping to rest and cool themselves along the way. And I knew that they took care of themselves in ways that we don't, because our concerns with the bottom line don't allow it."

The real question is whether the bottom line could indeed be impacted positively by allowing employees to have more control over the structure of their work schedule. It probably wouldn't work for those jobs where consistency of coverage and split-second timing are important. But not all work is like that. Particularly in information jobs, where workers' creativity and mental alertness determine the success of the endeavor, handcuffing people to a schedule that doesn't match their times of greatest concentration is in fact quite counterproductive.

Cognitive psychologist Pierce Howard agrees. In his book *The Owner's Manual for the Brain*, he tells you to chart your own needs for sleep, exercise, food, and so forth, and do whatever your body tells you it needs. He suggests such strategies as taking a twenty-minute walk to break up a long meeting or training session, and adjusting the lighting, visual distractions, and noise levels in work areas to match your own preferences. In other words, he warns managers and employees alike, it's critical to remember that one size *won't* fit all if you want people to be able to do their best work.[4]

Even high-powered business research is beginning to show that the hairy dogs do have something worth emulating. Researchers at

Stanford and Harvard business schools and McKinsey and Company, arguably the world's most prestigious training grounds for business leaders, have been coming to the shocking conclusion that paying attention to the needs and rhythms of individuals can enhance their productivity, and hence the effectiveness of the entire team. As Robert Waterman pointed out in *What America Does Right: Learning from Companies That Put People First*, when companies truly balance the needs of customers, shareholders, and employees—that is, when they listen to what their workers want—they are much more profitable than companies that think about customers and shareholders and ignore their own people.[5]

Arrangements like flex time and telecommuting go a long way toward allowing people to do their work in their own high-activity times rather than only between the hours of nine and five, at a specified place in the office. Managerial flexibility could also encourage employees to know their own "best times" and plan their own work accordingly whenever possible. It wouldn't be easy to make happen, but it would be invigorating to try. Managers who insist on regularity at all costs probably don't even know they're sacrificing creativity and innovation on the altar of consistency.

The question of natural rhythms is more than just an individual concern, however. There are some universal patterns as well. Research grounded in the Ayurvedic tradition of India reminds us that humans are the only species who don't have enough good sense to follow the natural circadian rhythms of each day. According to John Douillard and other Ayurvedic health-care practitioners, the daily routine that will best serve most of us is waking with the sun, or shortly thereafter; exercising and meditating in the morning; having a light breakfast; working hard until noon; setting aside at least an hour for a hearty and relaxing lunch, followed by a brief rest and a short walk; then working hard mentally from two to six p.m.; followed by a second meditation and a very light meal; ending the day with time quietly reading and bedtime before ten p.m.[6]

Of course, that might not work best for you—you'll have to observe yourself for a few weeks, preferably recording your observations in your career log, in order to get a sense of your own best rhythms. Once you have your own number, so to speak, then it's time to commit to a routine that fits you. One of the worst effects of career distress is falling into a *reactive* pattern of stumbling from one demanding, exhausting event into another, without a regenerative, organized routine to signal the beginnings and endings of your days.

"Right, sure I can take the time for morning meditation—you've gotta be out of your mind," gasped Caroline, management information systems director in a pharmaceutical firm, when I suggested that she might feel the stresses of her job less if she took more control of her daily routine and gave her body what it naturally needed. It seems, in fact, that corporate life has specifically been designed to violate every tenet of a healthy routine. The ways we (mal)adapt to it exacerbate the situation: jumping out of bed late and racing off to the office in a panic; then scarfing down a hurried lunch at your desk or at the drive-through. We often follow that with a heavy, fat-laden meal awash in alcohol late at night, and staying up into the early hours of the morning finishing a project or entertaining clients when our bodies want desperately to be resting and rejuvenating themselves for the next day. This is the deadly corporate dance that's making so many of us *feel terrible* and wonder why. And so what do we do about it? We take painkillers to dull the warning signals (there go the smoke detectors again) and keep on punishing ourselves.

Caroline was really in a bind. She loved her work, was making terrific money, and didn't want to leave, but it was clear from her physical state that something wasn't working. Corporate America is not about to have a conversion experience and turn into a health club, so if you, like Caroline, want to stay in a corporation because you enjoy the challenge and the perks there, you'll need to beef up your self-care strategies. Work toxicity is cumulative, like allergens—the higher the count, the more antidotes you need.

After her next bout with headaches and a sore throat, Caroline did accept my challenge to visit an Ayurvedic center to see if something could be done. There she learned about her particular body type and the foods and specific physical care her body naturally needed. The amazing part is that she analyzed her own natural rhythms and actually figured out ways to build into her schedule at least some of the life-balancing changes that were suggested to her. She was indeed able to add meditation, a morning walk, a longer and more relaxed lunch, and fewer late-night business meals to her "usual and customary" routine. She even feels her career has been enhanced, because she's feeling better and finishing projects with much more creativity and follow-through.

Eventually, some people decide there might be a link between how lousy they feel and what's happening at their work, so they come to talk about what other jobs they might be able to do. Many times, they are surprised to find out that they can stay in a job that feels toxic by adjusting their routine to be more congruent with both their own individual natural rhythms and the circadian rhythms that all species live by. It's up to you to figure out when and how you work best on individual tasks, when you're a little logy and need the stimulation of others, when you need to take a walk or do a brief meditation.

What Do You Have to Have?

There are several ways for people of even modest means to evade being trapped in an unrewarding career and to live more meaningful, more leisurely lives. All of them involve making decisions about what is essential and what can be discarded.   —BRAD EDMONDSON

What do you really need from your work? That's the essential question, and it's like your fingerprint—your answer won't be exactly like anyone else's. Nor will it stay the same for you over time. Each of you can figure out what you really need, by being honest with yourself and asking both your unconscious mind and your body to help you pull up information. The answers you'll get may surprise you. The following career wish list exercise is designed to help you assess work situations—past, present, or future—for how well they fit your needs, both the obvious ones and those obscured by the long shadow of practicalities and expectations.

CAREER WISH LIST EXERCISE

Step One: Digging Deep

It's often hard to pinpoint just why the work you're in just doesn't seem to fit anymore. I'd bet that most of you are not very practiced at ascertaining what you need in your work life—what skills you want to use the most, what the environment should be like, what meaning you'd like your work to have. The preparation stage of this exercise asks you to dig deep, setting aside time to ask yourself some probing questions. The more honest and thorough your answers are, the more helpful the exercise can be. Respond to the questions below with as many answers as you can imagine.

1. What skills and talents do you really enjoy using and/or want to develop more?

_____   _____

_____   _____

_____   _____

_____   _____

_____   _____

_____   _____

_____   _____

2. What features do you want in your work environment? Consider surroundings, perks, salary opportunities, schedules, organizational structures, and so forth.

_____   _____

_____   _____

_____   _____

_____   _____

_____   _____

_____   _____

_____   _____

3. What kinds of working relationships and supervisory style do you prefer?

_____   _____

_____   _____

_____   _____

_____   _____

_____   _____

_____   _____

4. What passions, values, interests would you like to be part of your work life?

_____ _____

_____ _____

_____ _____

_____ _____

_____ _____

_____ _____

Look over your responses to these four questions and circle or check off the *ten* that seem most critical. Then go back over the ten, rank them (10 = the most critical to you now), and list them on the chart below.

10 = _____ 5 = _____

9 = _____ 4 = _____

8 = _____ 3 = _____

7 = _____ 2 = _____

6 = _____ 1 = _____

Step Two: Checking the Fit

1. At the top of the checking-the-fit form opposite, write the title or a brief description of the opportunity you're analyzing.

2. Then, from your work-preference preparation pages, copy the list of your top ten essentials onto the left-hand column of the form. As you copy the items, double-check your answers and make any needed adjustments.

3. For each of the ten essential items in the left-hand column, estimate on a scale of 1 to 10, 10 being the best, how well you think that opportunity and that career essential fit with each other. Put your estimates in the middle column. Continue down the column until you've cross-referenced each of your essentials to this opportunity and given it a "goodness of fit" score.

4. Then, go back to the top of your form and multiply the number from the left-hand column by the quality of fit score in the middle column to get a "factor salience" score; enter that number into the right-hand column. Repeat this step for each of the ten essentials.

5. Finally, add all the numbers in the factor-salience (right) column to get a total "goodness of fit" score for the job or opportunity you're estimating. The total possible is 550.

Job/opportunity: _____

Essentials for a good fit	Quality of fit (1–10)	Factor-salience score
_____ 10 ×	_____ =	_____
_____ 9 ×	_____ =	_____
_____ 8 ×	_____ =	_____
_____ 7 ×	_____ =	_____
_____ 6 ×	_____ =	_____
_____ 5 ×	_____ =	_____
_____ 4 ×	_____ =	_____
_____ 3 ×	_____ =	_____
_____ 2 ×	_____ =	_____
_____ 1 ×	_____ =	_____

Total Goodness of Fit score   _____
for this opportunity   (550 possible)

The purpose of this preference exercise is to help you quantify and compare your needs with what's possible in the job you have or are considering. If the job you analyzed was worth less than 300 points for you, you'd be well-advised to ask yourself some hard questions. All too often I see people getting stuck in or rushing into opportunities or "hot jobs" that other people think are terrific for them, without digging deep enough into their own feelings and hunches. If you're surprised that you got such a low "fit" score for your present job, but aren't ready to leave, there are suggestions throughout the book that could let out some of the seams for you.

So Go and Get It!

I call intuition cosmic fishing. You feel the nibble, and then you have to hook the fish.   —BUCKMINSTER FULLER

You deserve to be in work that fits, because if you aren't, it will eventually make you sick. My client notes are chock full of stories about folks who made themselves ill by being afraid to ask if their jobs really worked for them, or too worn down to do anything about it.

"That's easy for you to say," Diane said in a shrill voice when I warned about the dangers of staying in her ill-fitting job.

"Tell that theory to my landlord and daycare person and the supermarket. This is reality we're talking here—not some magical tale of the job fairy, you know."

Diane did have a point. How could a thirty-seven-year-old single parent, with three kids turning in stellar performances of the terrible twos, isolated nines, and acting-out adolescent, dare to hope for work that fit? Turn the question on its head: How can she hope to survive and do justice to the parenting role she values so much if she's worn down emotionally and physically every day by going to do work she hates? The answer is, she can't. After Diane was hospitalized the second time for recurrent pneumonia, she figured that out. Then we were able to strategize in earnest.

The outcome of our strategizing and her researching and networking was actually very positive. In time, she was able to escape the prison of her job as a medical secretary, a position made all the more unbearable by the daily reminder that she had once been married to an anesthesiologist who decided he wanted to paint rather than practice medicine. So, he was making art guiltlessly and she was making herself sick.

Reluctantly, Diane agreed to do the career wish list exercise, just to run an audit of how well her "responsible" job was working for her. Digging out and ranking the ten essentials from her answers to the many questions was challenging. It had been a while since she had allowed herself to think about what she needed in her life, much less in her work.

Here's the list which eventually surfaced for Diane:

10 = Organizing events
9 = Change of pace/no regular routine
8 = Autonomy/freedom
7 = Writing
6 = Children's issues
5 = Friendly environment
4 = Laughter/humor
3 = Benefits–health insurance/making money
2 = Casual dress
1 = Time for out-of-doors activity each day

Does this sound like the profile of a mild-mannered and unassuming woman in white at the front desk? Obviously, it wasn't. Her score on the career wish list didn't break 200. Diane concluded that she couldn't tarry too long in her present job. Diane was an organizer by nature (her top choice) and so she got herself organized to do something about the results of this exercise. She contacted an old friend in the events-promotion field, who in turn set her up for a series of information interviews. She also worked at home on some articles about teaching health-maintenance skills to parents and kids. All the while, she was able to show up at the office each day knowing that an escape hatch was gradually opening. Within the year, after capitalizing on contacts in the health and wellness field and showing her portfolio of writing samples around, Diane landed a job as health-education events coordinator for a major HMO. It wasn't a perfect fit—her score was about 460. But she was confident that, after a while to get some good results, she'd be able to arrange some of the flexibility she wanted for herself, which would give her more time to be outdoors and to earn some additional money from her writing.

Like Diane, you have to take responsibility for keeping the fit of your job comfortable. It's not so hard really, once you get used to thinking this way.

7. Getting a Whole Life—Finally!

People don't grow old. When they stop growing, they become old. —DEEPAK CHOPRA

Getting older is really a gift, not only because it surely beats the only known alternative, but also because it requires you to pay more attention to how you're feeling, emotionally and physically. The signals just get louder and louder. But people ignore the *messages* their bodies are trying to give them because they interpret them as proof that they're aging. Our fearful notions about the effects of getting older stem from an earlier time. The life expectancy of babies born in the United States in 1900 was forty-nine years; for babies born in this decade, it is nearly eighty. It doesn't make any sense to be saddled with century-old expectations of being on the way out in your forties and fifties.

There is also no reason to put off learning how to have more conversations with your body about the things it knows you need. The attitude you bring to those talks with your body is a critical part of the balance you're seeking. Consider a seemingly bizarre approach like going to a quiet place and thanking your shoulders for the pain you're feeling there. Then ask them what advice they're trying to give you. If you haven't been on speaking terms with your body for a while (and the more work responsibility and tension you're carrying around with you, the more likely this is to be true), you need to speak slowly and softly and then *listen carefully* for a response.

Even die-hard cynics have been shocked at the body-to-self conversations they were able to have about what they should be doing for themselves.

It's Time to Play

Having a good time is the most neglected aspect of good health. —Julia Child

Start off, for instance, with some talk about combining work and play. "Something has to change," Ruthie said as she detailed the myriad infections she had endured over the past year. "I know my body is trying to tell me something, but I can't figure out what."

"Well," I prodded, "can you think back to what was going on when you had your first attack?" "Actually," she said, "something tells me it started just before my fifty-fifth birthday, when I began to think about the ten years I had left until retirement."

Ruthie had been a budget analyst and then comptroller for a hospital chain for much of her working life. She was bored, and often found herself wondering about starting her own business. But given the difference between her current salary and what she would be able to make on her own, Ruthie was contending with a serious case of golden handcuffs. Her husband, Don, a government supervisor, was under a doctor's care for hypertension. They had decided that they'd both stick it out in their boring jobs and plan for retirement.

"If we live that long," Ruthie added. Indeed, at the rate they were going, she had finally realized, they'd have very little physical or emotional vitality left by the time those magic years rolled around. And so, despite their lifelong commitment to playing it safe, at the urging of some friends who had come to me for a midlife turnaround, Ruthie and Don had decided to explore what other options existed for them. Even though they were not the type to have thought much about having fun at work, I asked them the standard career-counselor questions about what they could imagine doing for fun rather than for money. Not much response. Then I asked them a critical career-exploration question: "Whose work makes you jealous?" The same answer shot back from both of them: "Ruthie's brother George." "He's a veterinarian," Ruthie explained. "We'd really like to get paid for playing with animals." Then a cloud came over Ruthie's face: "But we're surely too old to go to veterinary school."

Such a common, knee-jerk reaction that was—presuming that enjoying animals means going to vet school, any more than wanting to include some writing in your job would mean becoming a novelist, or enjoying showing others how to do things would necessarily put you in a high school classroom somewhere. For some reason, most people persist in thinking of their careers as *photos* rather than *collages*, and miss opportunities to design composite careers combining many of their talents and passions.

Remembering the times I'd called over half the state trying to find pet care, I asked her about pet services. "How about something to do with training, kenneling, or grooming animals?" I asked. Little kids' grins flashed back at me: yes!

Now, this very practical couple did not decide overnight to leave their secure jobs to go off and play with animals. But they did begin researching various pet service business ideas. They also talked to brother George. As it turned out, he was indeed interested in supporting a kennel business, because his veterinary practice needed ancillary pet-care services. And so the venture was launched as a weekend sidecar to their regular jobs. Eventually they were able to cut back their work to part-time, and to engage George in helping them advertise their new venture through his practice. Within the year Don decided it was safe for him to quit and develop the new business full-time, while Ruthie stayed on at the hospital chain part-time to keep the health insurance and other benefits for the family. Slowly and carefully they built their pet-care center, and were able to play en route to "retirement" and beyond.

So Who Are You Really?

Acquiring self-knowledge is much more difficult to do than
to say, because most of us have been practicing just the opposite skill for so long.   —HARRY DENT, JR.

In addition to paying attention to your neglected passions, another piece of the puzzle for avoiding workplace toxicity in your
middle and later years is to keep a keen eye on your own evolving
value system. As you move into that never-never land of early middle age, your identity, not just as an achiever, but as a whole person,
becomes more important. Your age has a tremendous influence on
what motivates you. While consulting and conducting research at a
large corporation, for instance, I asked managers in the engineer-
ing unit what kinds of rewards they were looking for at work.
The differences in responses from one age group to another were
eye-opening.

Managers in their thirties said they were interested in getting
greater visibility and enhancing their reputation in the organization
or in their field. They wanted to work on special projects or task
forces so they'd be noticed by upper management. Folks in their forties were influenced more by money: salary and bonuses were the
critical elements for them. Managers in their fifties and beyond,
however, weren't primarily concerned with either of these. For
them, what mattered was flexibility in scheduling, to make space for
other things in their lives. They also wanted access to courses and
training in areas removed from their day-to-day work. They preferred situations where they could work very long hours on a project for a period of time, and then have time off to travel or do
something different before the next assignment. Despite the age differences, there were no differences in how committed or hardworking or successful any of these managers were. They just wanted
different rewards for their efforts.

In these interviews, workers were quite clear about the ways in
which their bodies let them know what they needed. And, as you
might expect, the older groups counted on those physical signals to
help them stay on course with their evolving values. How often do

you stop to ask what really motivates you now, as opposed to five, ten, fifteen, or thirty years ago, when you started working?

Many people are so taken up with success that they forget to pay attention to figuring out the meaning of what they are doing. This is what Doris, a single, six-figures public relations executive in her late fifties, told me when I asked her what she was proud of in her life. "To tell you the truth," she said, "in the cannibalistic world where I work, I figure I'm lucky to have a job at all. And when you add in the age factor, it gets to miraculous. So I've just not allowed myself to ask myself what I might have wanted to be doing to make a difference."

Luckily for Doris, recurrent back pain did get her to think about it. In fact, her bulging disc reminded her regularly that her life was devoid of passions. So she finally decided to take some action. With a friend who worked in events management, she explored organizations that seemed to have a social mission and that might benefit from some pro bono work. They enjoyed researching everything from homeless shelters to environmental advocacy groups. They finally settled on a children's hospital, and, after some networking to find out whom to approach, they offered their services to help with a newly launched capital campaign. The hospital was delighted, and welcomed Doris and her friend into the "family." When I asked Doris what she liked most about the experience, she grinned and said, "It was definitely being allowed to go down to the preemie ward and stroke the babies." Pretty soon she and her friend were regulars in the tactile kinesthetic volunteer group.

When I saw her next, Doris knew a lot about "touching therapy" for babies. She reported proudly that premature or sick infants who are stroked regularly grow and get well much more quickly than infants who don't. Talk about miraculous—Doris now had something outside herself and her demanding work life to find meaning in, and she hadn't had to leave her hard-to-replace job in order to get rid of the pain in her lower back.

Getting Older: Plum or Prune?

Human nature is neither good nor bad, but open to continuous transformation and transcendence.

—MARILYN FERGUSON

Some people do get older without getting wiser. In a sad interview for *Psychology Today* magazine, *Cosmopolitan* editor Helen
Gurley Brown observed that her last book, *The Late Show*, had not
been very successful. And is it any wonder? According to Brown,
it was "all about how I hate getting older." She said it best: "All I
can do is be very fearful that success is going to disappear pretty
soon, which it will because of how old I am. Isn't it a shame that
I just can't be thrilled and happy that I've had this wonderful magazine and terrific husband?"[1]

You've all seen older people filled with regret, longing, depression, and rage. Some expend tremendous energy desperately trying
to stop the clock. Others waste time blaming their ungrateful children or their abandoning spouse or their exploitative employer for
the things they couldn't have in life. I knew a woman in her eighties
who spent her last days in an exclusive nursing home cutting up all
the pictures of her children, grandchildren, and friends into smaller
and smaller pieces, to punish them for not being good enough to
her. This woman was self-centered, driven by appearances, and
judgmental even when she was in her thirties and forties. She
pushed many people away by her critical, biting comments and nar-
row prejudices. But throughout her life, no one had the courage to
tell her about herself, to urge her to try some different behaviors.
And so at the end, she sat, clearly caught in despair, weeping and
cutting.

An image that captures the dichotomy of possibilities in getting
older is the *plum* versus the *prune*. Fully developed people take on
the qualities of a plum: juicy, robust, brimming with sweetness to
share. They may become more frail physically, but that does not in-
terfere with their ability to embrace life. Many work past the min-
imum age for retirement, and then evolve into a pleasure-filled

schedule of unpaid work and service for the next fifteen or twenty years.

By contrast, people who become stagnant at midlife dry out and shrink like prunes. Sometimes they are quiet and bitter, and sometimes they bellow like wounded animals, thrashing out at a hostile universe. Their work, and their lives, are the enemy. One of the most important discriminators between plums and prunes is what their age means to them. In a country that worships youth and vilifies aging, it's often not easy to stay optimistic as you get older. Betty Friedan, in *The Fountain of Age*, sees the "mystique of age" as even more deadly than the "feminine mystique." She calls it "more terrifying to confront, harder to break through."[2] But plum people draw their energy from the spiritual conviction that getting older is a positive, natural, and even somewhat humorous process. They know that a changed appearance (as a friend of mine says, "when your bra size shifts from 34 B to 38 long") and a few physical inconveniences are a small price to pay for the wisdom and balance that only living half a century or more can bring. And so they aren't afraid of the inevitable.

One of the many good things that come from thinking about growing older is forcing some of our fears to the surface. One that I encounter frequently, particularly among women, is fear of poverty—the Bag Lady Syndrome. Incredible numbers of bright, talented women (Lily Tomlin and Shirley MacLaine among them) have confessed that at some deep level, they have expected to find themselves on the street someday. Why should this surprise anyone? All their lives, women have been told by the culture that they can't make it on their own, that they're somehow less valued and valuable than their brothers. They're even paid less for doing better work. So in many ways the Bag Lady Fear is a realistic reaction to the data women have osmosed from the atmosphere of their lives.

An analysis of a 1972 data set of twelve thousand high school seniors, both males and females, made by Clifford Adelman of the U.S. Office of Education is relevant here. Adelman looked at the data, which included things like SAT and GRE scores, undergraduate and graduate school grades, performance reviews throughout their careers, and self-reports of how well their studies and work fit together. This study was aptly titled *Women at Thirty-Something: Paradoxes of Attainment.* It discussed the incredible irony that the females surpassed the males on all measures of achievement except two: salary and expectations of promotion.[3] Is it any wonder that many women throughout their lives harbor fears about their ability to survive financially?

The problem with fear of poverty and fear of getting older is, of course, the insidious effect of that old law of self-fulfilling prophecy—over and over again, you keep on getting what you expect. That's both a psychological and spiritual law: we draw to us the things we fear the most. The baby boomers started turning fifty in 1995. By 2005 nearly half of the population will be over fifty. Imagine what will happen to worker productivity and health-care costs if they all buy into the prevailing images of decline and decay. So if you're a person with those fears playing in your head, understandable though they may be in this culture, you'd better be thinking of how to get them erased.

In fact, there is no reason for aging boomers to despair. Gerontologist Lydia Bronte interviewed 150 people ages 65 to 102 and discovered that more than half of them had had what they considered their most productive years *after age 50.* And more than a third said that their most important achievements happened *after age 65.*[4]

Keeping Your Balance: The VITAL Formula

We are all pilgrims on the same journey ... but some pilgrims have better road maps.   —NELSON DE MILLE

Staying healthy, happy, and productive all require that you learn to keep your psychological, physical, and spiritual balance. Lots of smart people are interested in the problems of unhealthy and unproductive workplaces and what to do about them. This has culminated in an explosion of body-mind, wellness, and "new management paradigms" literature over the past five years. You could probably take off a year or two from work to read it and not get through it all. The surprise is that, when you survey the separate literatures of *staying healthy* and *keeping people productive and creative*, you find the five ingredients of what I call the VITAL formula—Vision/Values, Intelligence, Touch/Training, Attitude, Love—on both lists, in one form or another. Unfortunately, the managers who lead us into corporate battle and the health-care professionals who treat the wounds we sustain there probably don't think much about the similarities, because they don't read each others' journals or books. So making the connection is up to you.

Let me share with you the VITAL formula, which I "prescribe" to help people keep tabs on all the parts of their lives on a regular basis. The five essential "whole life" ingredients are easy to remember when you use the acronym VITAL to carry them around with you. Some of the five VITAL elements actually happen at work. Others are linked less directly (but significantly) to what's happening for you on the job. Together they form a holistic system of self-care—you can't skimp on any of them for very long if you want to stay healthy and effective in your job.

In many organizations, a computer couldn't have done a more thorough job of designing cultural norms that are antithetical to these five essentials of health and productivity. That's obviously the bad news. The good news, on the other hand, is that some people are surviving and thriving in these environments—and you can too, if you really want to be there, and if you learn how to take care of yourself. Let's look at some of the prescriptions in each of the five VITAL areas.

Vision/Values: Believing in Your Work

You must have vision and a sense of purpose about your work. You also need a feeling of coherence and consistency between your work and your beliefs. The "sense of coherence" concept was developed by the late medical sociologist Aaron Antonovsky after World War II as he studied Holocaust survivors, trying to understand why some had fared so much better than others. He found that people who had a clear sense of the meaning of their lives and a strong spiritual or philosophical belief system were much more likely to stay healthy during traumatic times.[5] Since then many medical studies have confirmed that a purposeful life keeps you healthy. At the same time, many management studies have documented the important positive effects of motivating workers through teams organized around a strong commitment to their project.

If you are having trouble knowing whether your career and your beliefs are congruent, now is the time to make yourself think about it. Discord doesn't need to be *conscious* to do its physical and emotional damage. Meditation, journaling, tuning in to your dreams, and spending time alone outdoors all help you to plumb the depths of your own spiritual, social, and political values.

Obviously you need to decide whether you can believe in your organization or not—but your manager could probably be making it a lot easier. In vital, innovative organizations, leaders are meaning-makers. They translate the mission of the organization into easily understood, meaningful goals for employees at all levels. When they fail to do this, ennui is not far behind. The complaints reported back to me most frequently from bright, eager liberal arts graduates who have gone into the marketplace to find work they can believe in are "It's boring" and "It doesn't mean anything to me." Both are about the absence of passion at work.

The responsibility for Vision/Values falls on both sides of the table. Your manager needs to make it clear that the organization has a valuable mission. You, meanwhile, are obligated to stay self-aware and attuned to your own passions. Increasingly, workers are saying that "a good place to work" means even more than being treated well and challenged to grow. People who feel they are helping others report much better health and stay vital longer than people without a sense of altruism.[6] If an organization doesn't offer its people something they can believe in, then it can expect less than full productivity and more than a few sick days. Perhaps you've experienced that.

Some managers are excellent leaders—they know instinctively how to engender enthusiasm and commitment for a project. Others need help. If you find yourself working for a manager who seems to flunk cheerleading (or if you are one yourself), don't give up: the best antidotes to deficiencies in organizational zeal are probably right outside your door. Why not ask the people on your team what's important and exciting *for them* about the work you're all trying to do—and what they would imagine you could do together.

Here are some questions you could ask that can help you unearth a common vision:

- What parts of our mission as an organization seem most important to you?
- How do they mesh with your own personal beliefs and values?
- What things would you like to see us emphasizing more?
- What kinds of projects or programs would you particularly enjoy helping to launch or improve?
- How could our group be working together more effectively to help everyone get involved?

Ask the two or three people you know best to talk about these questions over lunch together. Once you get them excited too, you can decide how to get others to join in your conspiracy to bring more meaning to your department's work.

If the campaign to breathe more passion into the job isn't successful, then you have choices to make again. You can search for work that is closer to your core values and beliefs. Or you can follow the example of Doris, who found the meaning she longed to have by doing community service in the tactile kinesthetic therapy group. The only thing you *can't do* is forget about it.

Intelligence: Staying Challenged, Continuing to Learn

We're just beginning to see how important mental fitness and constant reeducation are to both emotional and physical well-being. Harvard professors are in the top percentile of oldsters in the United States. As University of California psychologist Howard Friedman wrote in the distinguished British medical journal *Lancet*, scientists, sometimes considered at risk for ill health because of their studiousness and somewhat antisocial ways, are actually the healthiest among us. Using a sample of senior citizens who had been identified as intellectually gifted during childhood, Friedman studied the relative survival rates of scientists and nonscientists. Nonscientists were 26 percent more likely to die in any given year than scientists. Moreover, 72 percent of scientists, but only 67 percent of nonscientists, reached age seventy. Since the sciences often require more ongoing, diligent study than other professions in order to keep current, something about continuous, challenging intellectual exercise seems to be good for us.[7]

Ongoing education—at work, in continuing-education courses, or in an actual degree-granting program—can protect you from several unhealthy factors. Bored people are more likely to be isolated, depressed, demoralized, and lacking in self-esteem. A 1984 study in an Irish medical journal, for instance, showed that lack of learning is as strong a predictor of cardiac disease as smoking and problems with blood pressure, weight, and cholesterol.[8]

Reading books, discussing ideas with your friends, or savoring the thrill of your favorite music or an art exhibit are all as important to your health and productivity as visiting the gym several times a week. When you make time for art and music, your cells vibrate with potential healing. Classical music is used to treat trauma, depression, and anxiety. It's even used to stimulate weight gain in premature babies. Music also enhances your ability to think and solve problems. In experiments at the University of California at Irvine, for instance, student IQ scores increased after listening to a Mozart piano sonata.[9] Intellectual and aesthetic stimulation enhances both your cardiovascular function and your resistance to infection.[10]

One of the most insightful observers of the workplace is Willis Harman, a futures researcher, strategic thinker, and president of the Institute of Noetic Sciences. Harman, who believes that Western industrial society is on the verge of major transformations, has this to say about the Intelligence ingredient:

Lifelong learning is the only kind of education that makes sense. Thus, the workplace can also be considered as a learning place. But the economy has difficulty adjusting to that idea. According to its rules, work is something you get paid to do, and education is something you pay for.[11]

Indeed, if we were really intent on applying what the research on preventive health is currently showing us, then continuing-education tuition, concert tickets, and art lessons would all be deductible under our flexible health benefits coverage.

Touch/Training: Tuning In to and Meeting Your Body's Needs

The key element for Touch/Training is its emphasis on being attuned to your body's signals—inviting internal conversations rather than obliterating messages with various anesthetics. This cluster of suggestions covers the alignment of physical and mental factors as a strategy for staying healthy enough to do your work well. Though some suggestions may seem on the surface to have little direct connection to your career, they are in fact critical to keeping you strong and highly functional at work.

We've experienced a revolution in health over the past several decades, as noninfectious disease nudged out infectious disease as our primary health problem. It's no longer epidemics that are doing us in, but rather our own behaviors, such as smoking, drinking too much, eating poorly, failing to exercise, trying to ignore our feelings, and losing ourselves in our work. A 1990 surgeon general's report, *Health 2000: Objectives for the Nation*, noted that nineteen of the twenty major causes of death and illness in the United States were *entirely lifestyle related.*[12]

Organizations can make it easy or hard for workers to stay in good physical shape. Long and exhausting schedules, required socializing over nutritionally bankrupt meals, and lack of access to fitness facilities are the obvious problems that employers often cause. Other less blatant but perhaps even more important ones have to do with creating an atmosphere in which mind and body are separate entities, and fun is the opposite of work. When work is deadly serious stuff, it's deadly all right—for individuals and organizations alike. Employers couldn't sustain these norms if they didn't have at least some implicit support from us in the trenches, however. I wonder how many of you are undercutting your achievement potential by "going along" with unhealthy practices, because the healthy ones require more effort and discipline.

Exercise, one of the most critical but neglected tonics available, is a great example of our often refusing to help ourselves. As one doctor I interviewed observed, "Exercise is a primary form of health care, not just a fitness option." Exercise increases your sense of well-being, which in turn enhances immune functioning, builds cardiovascular strength, and protects you against degenerative diseases such as diabetes, arthritis, and osteoporosis. It has also been proven to combat anxiety, depression, sleep problems, and panic attacks. Most experts suggest three different kinds of exercise for maximal health enhancement:

- Stretching, for flexibility
- Aerobics, such as jogging, swimming, or walking, for cardiovascular efficiency
- Strength training, with weights or resistance machines, to strengthen muscles, connective tissue (tendons and ligaments), and bones and enhance central nervous system functioning

Exercise is tricky to recommend—because so many people view it as a necessary evil. Remember that perception is everything: so how you think about your exercise will probably determine whether you continue it and how positive the effects are. If you want exercise to work for you, it's important to choose a form, a setting, and a time that will let it feel like fun and "being good to yourself." Eventually the feeling you get will keep you doing it. "I couldn't endure the stress of my job if I didn't get to exercise it away in the gym after work," one executive told me.

"Time out" is another Touch/Training tonic that people often refuse. A study by the marketing unit for Hilton Hotels reported in

1995 that 38 percent of the people they interviewed had not taken any vacation in more than a year. Twenty-seven percent were nervous about their work while on vacation, and 19 percent said they couldn't stop thinking about it. Thirteen percent actually took work along with them. Most people who have taken time away (even when they didn't think they needed it) have reported on their return that they didn't know how exhausted they had been. Many have confided to me that they hadn't realized how much they were shortchanging the organization by not taking time to renew. Whenever the renowned psychologist Carl Jung was about to begin writing a new book, for instance, he would go to the beach and play in the sand, making passages for water to swirl and flow in different directions. He did this to gain access to the childlike creativity of his unconscious, in order to write with as much vitality and depth as possible. How many of you strategize in that way about tapping into your own achievement power?

Laughter and fun should also be on your preventive medicine shelf. Studies at UCLA, Stanford, and other institutions show that laughter protects against disease and enhances healing. It reduces immune suppressors as well as the stress hormones epinephrine and cortisol, and speeds up the production of immune system enhancers, such as beta-endorphins. Hearty laughter is also good exercise: one hundred hearty laughs is equal to ten minutes of rowing. Robust laughter speeds the heart rate, accelerates breathing, and increases oxygen consumption, all of which are great for your cardiovascular system.

Stanford psychiatrist William Fry has noted that laughter involves first a period of vigorous exercise of the muscles of the face, shoulders, diaphragm, and abdomen, followed by the experience of relaxation. He surmises that the combination of arousal and relaxation is what makes laughter such a good antidote to heart disease, depression, and other stress-related conditions. Evidently hospitals believe in humor: many now have laughter rooms or humor carts, stocked with fake noses and glasses, toys, joke books, and other things to make patients chuckle. Humor is also showing up with increasing frequency as a topic for management-development seminars—it's fun to imagine what form the first Fortune 500 humor cart might take!

You also need physical touch—in relationships, massage therapy, or through massaging your own body with oils or lotions. Physical stimulation releases healing growth hormones into the immune system. Americans have physical contact with each other much less than people in other cultures; only in England do people touch less than we do. We pay for that lack of tactile stimulation in diminished immune system effectiveness. Willingness to try new tactile stimulation strategies does sometimes turn up in unusual places, however. In an article called "The Knead Is Great," James Hirsch wrote of an increasing use of on-site massage in corporations. The massage takes place in conference rooms, where employees relax in massage chairs. Some organizations, confident that the therapeutic touch releases stress and improves productivity, pay for part of the massage therapist's fee.[13]

In my own busy office at Smith College, where staff members are on the front lines responding to demands all the time, we import both a massage therapist and a yoga teacher to work with staff during the highest-stress periods of our year. We always do our work with much more energy for several days after a massage or yoga session. We also keep a thirty-six-inch-diameter bright blue "physioball" right by the reception desk, inviting stressed-out job seekers of all ages to bounce or roll around on it and massage themselves for a few minutes while they wait to see a counselor. You wouldn't believe the soothing effect for those who are uninhibited enough to try it!

Sleep is critical also. Economist Juliet Schor estimates that most Americans are getting sixty to ninety minutes less sleep than they need each night. Fatigue creeps up on you when you're stressed at work and destroys your body's ability to cope with challenges and resist illness. Lack of sleep also interferes with dreaming, which is critical to both physical and emotional rejuvenation. Your unconscious mind works out many of your conflicts in dreams, and generally prepares you for the challenges of the day. Schor's observation: "If you need an alarm clock, you're probably sleeping too little."[14]

Eating well is obviously essential, too. Of course you know you need low-fat, low-cholesterol, low-sodium meals, with emphasis on grains, fruits, and vegetables, in order to give your body the fuel it needs to do the work you want it to do. But how possible is that, when your work is organized around meetings and events featuring elegant, high-fat meals or when it seems like there's only time for fast-food take-out or pizza? Most health experts also stress regular, moderate-sized meals, eaten sitting down, and your paying careful attention to when your body has had enough. They tell you to resist the temptation to eat on the run, because you can't perceive your body's responses to food when you're traveling at high speed. The aim is chewing slowly, thoroughly, letting your body savor the full taste of every mouthful. Food that is bolted, rather than chewed carefully, leaves you unsatisfied and, ironically, much more likely to overeat. How well does this square with the fact that one out of every six American meals is eaten in a car?

Vitamin awareness, intentional planning for meeting daily nutritional needs from food alone or a combination of food and supplements, is also part of staying healthy. It's estimated, by the way, that only 20 percent of Americans get the nutrients they need to stay vital. People are often amused when I begin career consultations asking about how well they've been treating their body lately—but you won't have the energy you need to make career changes unless you're taking good care of your body.

Another important Touch/Training strategy has to do with various forms of relaxation response and meditation. Jon Kabat-Zinn, Joan Borysenko, and other pioneers in what has become known as behavioral medicine have proven again and again that conscious relaxation and meditation strategies improve the body's cardiovascular and immune-system functioning. Transcendental meditation, introduced to the United States by Maharishi Mahesh Yogi in 1959, has been shown to reduce metabolism by 16 percent, while sleep reduces it by 12 percent. Therefore, meditation is more regenerative than sleep—and you can do it almost anytime, anywhere.

I know one corporate consultant who uses meditation to keep his mind clear and fight fatigue and stress as he jostles about in strange cities. He often pulls off the road in his rental car en route to a meeting to meditate for twenty minutes and rejuvenate himself. He learned TM in the late sixties, when thousands of people began using meditation to manage stress and improve their mental and physical well-being. The movement has been expanded and generalized even more in the past decade, as practitioners of behavioral medicine have documented the linkages between good health and the ability to find regenerative stillness inside yourself.

Lianne, a physician, should have known better than to ignore the Touch/Training imperatives. She'd been working fourteen to sixteen hours a day for more than a year, getting her family medicine practice up and running. She'd suggested slowing down to her two partners, both men, but they'd been unwilling to listen. Now there was no choice. She had just been diagnosed with rheumatoid arthritis, and, if they didn't want to lose her, they'd be forced to collaborate on different arrangements for managing the practice.

You'd think Lianne could have figured out for herself what she might be doing to her body with her relentless work demands and no time to do the things she needed to do, but the medical culture was a critical factor in her case. Medical people pride themselves on being able to withstand killer routines, and those who refuse to conform often find their competency called into question. In fact, one hospital now developing a stronger stress management program is doing so in response to the sudden cardiac death of their star chief resident in surgery, a thirty-three-year-old male. So it's no wonder that Lianne, who was already swimming upstream against the cultural assumption that women can't hold their own in medicine, almost worked herself into a state of collapse. Once she had her diagnosis of rheumatoid arthritis, however, another part of her kicked in. She helped her doctor with devising a regimen for her: a gentle exercise routine, a special diet, a schedule of alternating office hours and reading time, and the installation of a sauna at home. As for the partners in her practice, they had to agree to a more gradual plan for building the practice. Their families were delighted. So it turned out that everybody benefited from Lianne's encounter with her body's message system.

One final but critical aspect of Touch/Training is body image. Continually feeling bad about how your body looks limits your self-esteem, which eventually undercuts your immune power. Feeling physically weak or out of shape also wears away your sense of personal efficacy. Both of these engender a pervasive feeling of low-level stress, which, when exacerbated by another sudden stressful event, can contribute to artery blockages, blood platelet clumping, and sudden cardiac arrhythmias. Do you think you're giving away some of your personal power by underestimating your own attractiveness and self-sufficiency?

I remember a life-changing interaction with my own therapist some years ago, when we were discussing how I felt about my body and appearance. She asked me to gather up old photographs of myself which I liked and bring them to our next session. Reluctantly but dutifully, I arrived at her office with a large manila envelope full of photos. Together, we looked carefully at each of the old photographs. "In this one of you at age twenty-six, at your brother's wedding," she asked, "how do you think you looked?"

"Okay," I said. "Better than I remember."

She nodded, and went on. "And this one with the kids in Florida at age thirty?"

I hesitated. "Well, not bad. That was a pretty good haircut." And on she proceeded with eight or ten other photographs.

Then came the critical question. "And how did you feel *then* about your appearance? Did you let yourself know then that you were not so bad-looking?"

Both of us knew the sobering answer. Like so many of my own clients, I had dragged along with me from my adolescence a propensity to be extraordinarily critical of my own body. It was not the body that needed changing that much; it was the lens of the beholder.

The most important thing my therapist had to say came next. She said, "I want you to go home tonight and take a good look at yourself in the mirror, fully clothed. Take whatever time you need to look with appreciation at what you see there. Then, when what you're seeing looks good, take off your clothes and look some more. Resist the tendency to look away or wish you were different. Look with approval and affection at the curves of your middle-aged body. *Because this is as good as it gets.* Why wait ten or twenty years again, when you've drifted even more and have hundreds of new wrinkles, to appreciate *in retrospect* how you look today?"

Her message was tricky, but clear. By all means, find a way in your overstuffed life to give your body the exercise, rest, and good nutrition it needs to stay strong, but *don't* be disapproving of how it looks. You need to like yourself to stay healthy.

Attitude: Feeling Optimistic and In Control

People who feel little sense of control over their personal or professional lives fall prey to higher rates of accidents, depression, and physical illness. So pervasive is the effect of attitude on health that J. M. T. Finney, a professor of surgery at the Johns Hopkins Medical School, stated in 1934 that he wouldn't operate on people who entered surgery believing they wouldn't survive the operation. Finney knew even then that "what you expect is what you get."[15]

Many people first notice they're depressed or anxious when their work becomes less and less enjoyable. Career complaints can be a flag for career counselors and family members alike to consider that a person should be assessed for depression, anxiety, or some other emotional problem for which trained psychological help is required. If you are clinically depressed, you can't will away your sadness— you need medical treatment. You should consult a health-care practitioner as quickly as possible. For most of us, however, positive thinking and self-awareness can be learned.

Hopefully, you're committed to understanding your own behavior as honestly as possible, to keeping an open mind about things, and to adjusting your judgments as new information comes to you. And do you enjoy the challenge inherent in changing the way you do things from time to time? If you and several people who know you well agree that the answers to these questions for you is yes, then your immune system is probably strong, say most body-mind researchers. It's a modern example of better living through chemistry. When you're afraid to really look at yourself and resist change, your body produces cortisol, a deadly stress hormone. But when you're excited and eager about what's ahead, your internal apothecary produces interleuken-2, the magic growth substance currently used to treat cancer and other immune system breakdowns. I've found over the years, however, that few of us are very good at perceiving our own negativity—it usually has to be pointed out to us. Just to be sure, screw up your courage and ask a few people at home and work how often your thoughts have a negative tinge. Then be prepared to do something about what you hear.

It's also sickening to feel unequal to the tasks facing you at work. In a study of 139 corporate managers, matched for age, sex, income, diet, and heredity, one factor seemed to predict who got sick. Those managers who had risen to their current positions without a college education felt less secure and more threatened—and fell sick much more often than their more credentialed colleagues.[16] If you find yourself devaluing yourself because you feel less educated or less able than your co-workers, check it out with your supervisor. Ask her directly if your performance is less adequate than your peers'. If she says no, then the work is internal: get some help bringing your negative chatter more into line with what's real. If she says yes, then a different kind of next move is in order. Find out what training or education you need, and get started, one little step at a time. The one thing not to do is worry in silence, making yourself sick and compromising your performance.

One final observation about feeling in control is that it's often hard to hold on to your confidence during a job search—it seems as if it's an employers' market and as if employers have got you dangling on a string. In this situation, many people fall into a passive, reactive mode, dutifully applying for jobs in the newspaper, knowing there will be hundreds of equally qualified applicants. And so they wait for the ax to fall, wondering why they get more depressed and sick. It's critical to *take control* of the situation in any way you can—doing research, arranging information interviews, networking with various people in your own and related fields, offering your services on a pro bono basis, and so forth, while you try to crack that "hidden job market" or create a position for yourself. Remember that most of the jobs lost in the past decade have been replaced with new and different ones. But the new ones are seldom in the paper—you'll have to network and scramble to find them. Staying active will keep you well, as you think about next steps or even as you endure a harrowing period of unemployment; waiting passively for a prince of a job to show up in the classifieds will make you ill.

Love: Expressing Feelings and Building Relationships

Research says quite clearly that staying healthy requires staying in touch with your feelings and taking good care of your relationships. It's no accident that lonely people are sicker and more likely to die than their counterparts in meaningful relationships of one kind or another. Negative biological reactions, such as the weakening of your immune capability and cardiovascular stress, occur during separations or disruptions from loved ones. They also occur in the presence of people with whom you have stressful relationships. Researchers found when testing married couples that disagreeing lowered their measured levels of infection-fighting NK and T cells.[17] If you're arguing a lot with people at home or at work, your immune system is probably pretty unhappy about it.

But sexual partnerships are not the only relationships that can help to keep you strong. Fortunately, good friendships can create the same joy and feeling of being understood—without some of the hassles inherent in merging two lives.

Relationships that are one-sided, limited in the expression of genuine affection, unable to withstand real differences of opinion, or pushed aside repeatedly in deference to career demands don't have the same healing, sustaining qualities as full, rich ones. Both single people and unhappily married people report poorer health than people who are happily married or partnered.

Extended family connections are also potentially health-preserving. A study of a tight-knit enclave of Italian Americans in Roseto, Pennsylvania, showed the degree to which emotions can modulate other factors. What was remarkable about this community was the unexpected discrepancy between their diets, which were very high in fat, and their cardiovascular health, which remained excellent. The researchers concluded that the supportive atmosphere of the extended family had been sufficient to counterbalance the effects of the questionable diets.

The story didn't end there, however. Over time the family ties began to weaken, as younger members of the family pulled back, moved away, and generally invested much less of themselves in the extended family. As this change in the family culture evolved, the heart disease rates for the community escalated, and within a period of years began to equal the national norms for cardiovascular disease.

Relationships even make a difference with animals, it seems. In experiments testing the relationship between high-fat diets and artery disease, one group of rabbits developed less atherosclerosis than the other groups, even though they were being fed the same high-fat meals. This finding perplexed the research team until they discovered that their population of rabbits was being tended by a medical student who was short, and who could reach into only those cages on the bottom tier of rows of cages stacked several high. The student had formed a relationship with the rabbits she could reach and accompanied their feeding with petting and talking to them. This was enough to slow the onset of their disease.

Having pets at home has also been shown to be vitalizing. In study after study, researchers have found that people who have pets stay healthier. Animals give you a sense of being needed. They also show you how to play, to put aside your work stresses, and to enter the realm of the absurd with some of their antics. Sometimes they take you on walks or out into nature. And they think *you* are wonderful! Each of those factors has been shown to be a major health enhancer.

Putting VITAL to Work

So what do you do with this understanding of the VITAL formula? How do you put it to use in daily practice? Perhaps Molly can show you how. Molly brought with her from her girlhood in the South a dramatic nature and a love of excess: the more rich foods, the more parties, the more luxurious entertaining, the more hazardous brushes with deadlines, the more energized she felt. Life on the edge was exhilarating to her. And it seemed to work for her, until she turned forty-two and was promoted to director of marketing for a major nonprofit organization.

In her new role, she needed to be more steady, less self-absorbed and impulsive, and an aware and reliable resource to the team who reported to her. Gradually it became obvious that Molly's old ways of ricocheting from one challenge to another wouldn't work in this new role. She had come up short on several major long-term projects and was feeling terrible, physically and emotionally, much of the time. That's when she came to see me about possibly needing to change jobs again.

After some discussion about the pace of her life, I suggested that she take the *Career Vitality Inventory*, an assessment tool based on the VITAL formula which I use in counseling sessions, as a check on the compatibility of the various systems in her life. Perhaps you can predict the results. Molly's score on Vision/Values was off the scale—she believed in what she was doing, and she was committed to her organization's mission. That's why the thought of leaving had been so devastating. Her score on Love was high also, because she had continued to commit real time to her relationships. Her Attitudes score was in the middle, but had slipped somewhat, she felt, based on how things seemed to be so out of control at the moment. Whereas she had once felt confident, now she felt unsure of herself in this new role. It surprised her to find out that Intelligence was below average, because so much of the job was new. But when she considered it more carefully, it was clear that she had been in such a fast-forward, reactive mode that her real learning had slowed down, just at the moment she needed it most. She was bouncing from crisis to crisis and not taking in much. What was really depressing, as you might imagine, was her Touch/Training score. Here she was flunking badly.

We carefully worked out a system that she was willing to follow to get herself in better physical balance. Then she could get to the business of deciding whether the new job might be manageable and enjoyable, if she were giving herself the benefit of her new daily practice.

In fact, Molly did decide to stay with the director's job, after she learned how to be in the driver's seat in her own life. Here's what she decided to put into her individually designed practice:

- A daily half-hour walk on a newly purchased treadmill.
- Deep breathing for twenty minutes each day.
- A yoga class one night a week with a friend.
- The purchase of several exciting heart-smart cookbooks to help her counterbalance the required business lunches with healthy suppers at home.
- A weekend executive-education program with particular training in strategic marketing.
- A brief therapy contract for eight sessions at her HMO, to figure out what her lifelong compulsion to "go fast" might be about.

It took several months, but Molly started to feel very differently about her work. She felt in control of her own life. She had much more energy and was able to plan and execute long-term projects successfully. In therapy, she saw her "life on the edge" style for what it had been, a way to stay hyped-up through activities and demands and to run away from her own long-buried sad and fearful thoughts, at great physical cost to herself. Had she just decided to leave the new job without taking a harder look at the ways in which she needed to have this new *daily practice* in place, she would inevitably have played out the same scene in her new position.

Create a Positive Plot

The number one managerial objective in most big firms
should be creating a revolution. —JOHN KOTTER

Clearly, individuals have to take responsibility for using the VI-
TAL formula to detoxify their own work. But it goes much easier
when employees and organizations work together on the problem.
Thus the suggestion for a "vital conspiracy"—a systematic coming
together of workers and their leaders, who have so often stared
menacingly at each other across the fence of disparate agendas.
When you act alone, you can be true to your own values and needs,
which is very important. But you never get as much leverage as you
can from joining forces with others to make your place of employment as vital as possible.

Such boundary-breaking collaborations are seldom easy, as Jack
Welch found out at General Electric. In the eighties, as a new CEO,
Welch engineered sweeping changes at GE—massive restructuring,
selling off business units that didn't dominate in their own mar-
kets, and a revolutionary commitment to breaking up hierarchies and
reeducating the entire workforce. Welch encountered resistance at
every turn: people seemed determined to languish in comfortable
roles rather than risk trying potentially exciting new things.

Other corporations report similar pockets of resistance and sabotage. Though middle managers are most often blamed for obstruct-
ing change, senior executives and line workers also get in the way
of proposed organizational transformations. As one human resources manager in a manufacturing firm told me, "People are
amazing. They may tell pollsters they're willing to trade salary for
better quality of life and more free time, but if anyone says a word
about limiting their overtime, they howl." It would be safe to say
that people at all levels are conflicted, about whether organizations
are capable of changing enough to be health-enhancing rather than
toxic and about how many alterations in their own habits and assumptions they're willing to make.

Management also sets the tone that tells workers whether it's safe to bring their feelings into the office. Fortunately, some people high up in quite visible organizations are beginning to notice that there might be some relationship between access to feelings and workers' effectiveness. Management consultant Noel Tichy, in his compelling description of the revolutionary changes executed at General Electric by Jack Welch, had this to say about emotions and work:

> Work, inevitably, is an emotional experience; healthy people can't just drop their feelings off at home like a set of golf clubs. Yet management theory long neglected this realm, and we are just beginning the search for ways to harness the vast power of workers' emotional energy.[18]

Because many organizations can't tolerate real emotions at work, there is little room for honest exchanges, which almost always involve some degree of anger, disappointment, jealousy, or hurt feelings in the "working through" process. What if you tried to run your friendships or your family without any real displays of emotion—what dishonesty would be required! And how much less vital they would be. Organizations need people who can pick up on signals and communicate effectively, both of which require our antennae to emotional issues to be functioning well. We don't let color-blind people become spies or pilots for fear they'll miss important signals. So why do we let feelings-impaired people manage organizations and miss critical emotional information all the time? Particularly when the most important conversations needing to be had by managers and workers are ones about how to anticipate, acknowledge, and draw on each other's feelings in response to the pressures and opportunities in organizational life today.

Despite unprecedented numbers of articles, books, and trainings about quality management, worker empowerment, and team-building, many organizations are still a war zone of managers versus employees. In addition, employees are often locked into combat with each other for a shrinking supply of rewards, and even jobs. The need for sensitive and skillful leadership to enable people to work together in vital conspiracies has never been greater than it is now. As Mitch Rabkin, president of Beth Israel Hospital in Boston, quipped in a keynote address to the New England Business for Social Responsibility conference, "Being a manager these days is tantamount to practicing psychiatry without a license."

Positive conspiracies between bosses and the bossed are all the more important now, because in most organizations going to work has become like living in California or Florida—earthquakes and storms are just part of the deal. Nobody can know when somebody's currency will take a tumble and affect you, when a competitor will upstage your company's most critical product, or when new legislation will totally upend your way of doing business. The most people-oriented CEO in the world couldn't take away the anxiety-producing turbulence of the global marketplace, any more than the governors of those two states could stop natural disasters from happening. But there are things that individuals, organizations, and governments have learned to do to make life less hazardous there. The VITAL formula is not just for individuals. Making a commitment to implementing it at work, as both an individual and an organizational strategy, could help make your workplace feel more disaster-resistant.

How could organizations create environments that would make it easier for workers to use the VITAL system? And how healthy is the place where you work? Look at the list below, and check which health-enhancing policies and practices are already in place in your organization.

Vision/Values

____ A clear organizational mission communicated effectively to employees: something for workers to believe in

____ Mutual trust between managers and workers

____ A clear mandate from the top to value workers

____ Opportunities for employee involvement in fine-tuning and implementing the goals of the organization

____ Top-down commitment to cultural diversity and affirmative action—guaranteed full inclusion for older, minority, female, gay, disabled workers

Intelligence

____ Commitment from the top for ongoing organizational change and new learning

____ Accessible, high-quality employee training and development programs at all levels

____ Tuition-reimbursement programs

____ A strong commitment to honest feedback up, down, and around in the organization

____ A career development program available to each employee, individually and in groups

Touch/Training

____ A policy in support of using vacation time and taking weekends and holidays for leisure, regeneration, and relationships

____ Acceptance of individuality and playfulness at work—in dress, scheduling, and approaches to tasks

____ Encouragement to laugh and have fun on the job

____ Accessible fitness facilities and encouragement to employees to schedule physical activities into the work week—lunchtime walks, yoga, early-morning or after-hour aerobics, and so forth

____ Organizational support for meditation, relaxation training, massage, or other body-mind stress interventions

Attitude

____ Clear performance goals and an ongoing, effective feedback system to let employees know how well they're meeting expectations

____ Employee involvement in redesigning tasks and organizational structure, to build a sense of worker responsibility and control

____ Self-directed work teams

____ Supportive, non-blaming, respectful management styles; upbeat, optimistic atmosphere

____ Procedures in place for employees to give supervisors feedback about their managerial effectiveness

Love

_____ Permission for employees to express their thoughts and feelings without fear of retribution

_____ An effective employee assistance program

_____ Access to flex time, telecommuting, and other flexible ways to get work done when necessary

_____ Adequate personal days and health-care days to enable employees to meet their obligations to their families

_____ Permission for employees to be "whole people" at work, expressing emotions and sharing their personal lives with co-workers

So how did your organization score on this mini-quiz? Hopefully, the test items gave you some ideas about where to begin with your positive plot.

What a great setting for a vital conspiracy: a turbulent economic drama in which employees and organizations both need something from each other. Workers obviously need their jobs. Contrary to media portrayals of workers as expendable, most organizations also want to hold on to a cadre of healthy, productive employees who have learned to work well together. It's _expensive_ to find and train talent.

Remember this—you are not only affected by your work environment. You are also remaking the energy there all the time by your own reactions and interactions with others. If you can get enough people involved in changing the assumptions and the atmosphere of the place, as well as their interactions with each other, then you could see much of the toxicity abate.

Joline Godfrey, author of _Our Wildest Dreams: Women Entrepreneurs Making Money, Having Fun, Doing Good_, has this to say about what's possible in organizations in which managers and employees have found ways to become co-conspirators:

Fun companies are full of alive, vital people. They have a gleam in their eyes—a sense of mischievous daring about them. The air around them is often electrified. . . . Industry is palpable. Just below the surface is the life force that keeps it happening. Inherent in that life force is a large element of playfulness and adventure. Isn't this fun? Isn't this grand? Aren't we lucky to be on this wonderful adventure?[19]

You Can Be Your Own Canary

> The people who get on in this world are the people who get up and look for the circumstances they want, and, if they can't find them, make them. —GEORGE BERNARD SHAW

In her book *When the Canary Stops Singing: Women's Perspectives on Transforming Business*, Pat Barrentine recalls the story of using canaries in the coal mines, as a signal to the miners that the air had become toxic. When the canaries stopped singing, the miners knew it was time to get out of there. Hopefully, you have learned to listen to your body and your emotions telling you when something's not right, long before you stop singing.

Some people wait until their life is close to over before they begin asking what it has been all about and what they might have done differently. Then, when their bodies try to help out by sending them some signals, they conclude they're being picked on. "My body hates me," one woman in her forties used to say over and over, recounting the unpleasant symptoms she felt when she was eating poorly, sleeping too little, and trying to cram a month's project into a week. So she took painkillers and pressed on, while her body was saying in every way it could, "Stop this nonsense."

You can wait until you're older, if you wish, or you can start now to listen better. You have not only my *permission* but also my *strongest encouragement* to have a "whole life" right now. Your body will help, your family, friends, and colleagues will help—and you'll all be better for the effort. You can transform your discomfort into the determination you need to choreograph the career and life your mind, spirit, and body want you to have.

You'd be surprised how many people are content with half a life or less—and they often use workplace toxicity as an excuse for not going after what they want, at work or in their personal lives. "I'm too busy." "I can't afford it." "I don't feel well enough to do that." But now the jig is up: in *Toxic Work* you've seen that there's no need to settle for less than you deserve. You can manage the stressors, and you can find the opportunities in the problems.

Author Marilyn Ferguson observed, "No one can persuade another to change. Each of us guards a gate of change that can only be opened from inside. We cannot open the gate of another, either by argument or emotional appeal." Hopefully, you'll decide *now* to swing open that gate for yourself, to begin to experience a new, whole life.

NOTES

Introduction

1. L. Dossey. *Meaning and Medicine: Lessons from a Doctor's Tales of Breakthrough and Healing.* New York: Bantam, 1991.

2. *Work in America: Report of a Special Task Force to the Secretary of Health, Education, and Welfare.* Cambridge, Mass.: MIT Press, 1973.

Chapter 1: The Toxic Workplace

1. Smith College, July 1991, Senior Administrative Management Seminars, and subsequent conversation.

2. David Noer. *Healing the Wounds: Overcoming the Trauma of Layoffs and Revitalizing Downsized Organizations.* San Francisco: Jossey-Bass, 1993.

3. Attributed to Senator Thomas A. Daschle, Congressional Record, April 2, 1993.

4. L. Dossey. *Meaning and Medicine: Lessons from a Doctor's Tales of Breakthrough and Healing.* New York: Bantam, 1991, p. 83.

5. Robert Waterman. *What America Does Right: Learning from Companies That Put People First.* New York: W. W. Norton, 1994.

6. Juliet Schor. *The Overworked American: The Unexpected Decline of Leisure.* New York: Basic Books, 1992.

7. Todd Erkel. "Time Shifting," *The Family Therapy Networker*, January–February, 1995, pp. 33–39.

8. R. Barnett. "Home-to-Work Spillover Revisited: A Study of Full-Time Employed Women in Dual-Earner Couples," *Journal of Marriage and Family* 56 (3), 1994, pp. 647–56. Also in discussion and conversation at the Nag's Heart conference, Amherst, Mass., June 1995.

9. P. Capelli, J. Constantine, C. Chadwick. *It Pays to Value Family: Work and Family Trade-Offs Reconsidered*. Philadelphia: Center for Human Resources at the Wharton School, University of Pennsylvania, 1995.

10. Stephen Covey. *The 7 Habits of Highly Effective People: Powerful Lessons in Personal Change*. New York: Simon and Schuster, 1989.

11. Marvin Weisbord. *Productive Workplaces: Organizing and Managing for Dignity, Meaning, and Community*. San Francisco: Jossey-Bass, 1991.

12. Margaret Wheatley. *Leadership and the New Science: Learning About Organization from an Orderly Universe*. San Francisco: Berret-Koehler, 1993.

13. Blair Justice. *Who Gets Sick: How Beliefs, Moods and Thoughts Affect Your Health*. Los Angeles: Jeremy P. Tarcher, 1987.

14. Robert Karasek. *Healthy Work: Stress, Productivity, and the Restructuring of Working Life*. New York: Basic Books, 1992.

15. Ellen Langer and Susan Saegert. "Crowding and Cognitive Control," *Journal of Personality and Social Psychology* 35(3), pp. 175–82.

16. Rosabeth Kanter. *When Giants Learn to Dance: Mastering the Challenge of Strategy, Management, and Careers in the 1990s*. New York: Simon and Schuster, 1989.

17. G. L. Engel and A. H. Schmale. (1972) "Conservation-Withdrawal: A Primary Regulatory Process for Organismic Homeostasis." CIBA Foundation Symposium 8, *Physiology, Emotion and Psychosomatic Illness*. Amsterdam, Holland: Associated Scientific Publishers.

18. Blair Justice. *Who Gets Sick*. p. 72.

19. S. Maddi and S. Kobasa. *The Hardy Executive: Health Under Stress*. Chicago: Dorsey Professional Books, Dow-Jones-Irwin, 1984.

Chapter 2: Just How Toxic Is Your Work?

1. Dean Ornish. *Stress, Diet, and Your Heart: A Lifelong Program for Healing Your Heart Without Drugs or Surgery*. New York: Signet, 1984, p. 50.

2. W. Whitehead. "Gut Feelings: Stress and the G.I. Tract," in D. Goleman and J. Gurin (eds.), *Mind/Body Medicine*. New York: Consumer Reports Books, 1993, p. 171.

3. J. Kabat-Zinn. *Full Catastrophe Living*. New York: Delacorte, 1990.

4. Goleman and Gurin (eds.). *Mind/Body Medicine*.

5. Murray Mittleman. "Triggering of Myocardial Infarction Onset by Episodes of Anger," *Circulation* 89, 2 (1994).

6. S. G. Haynes. "Type A Behavior, Employment Status, and Coronary Heart Disease in Women." *Behavioral Medicine Update* 6 (4), pp. 11–15.

7. U. Lundberg. "Urban Community: Crowdedness and Catecholamine Secretion," *Journal of Human Stress* 2, pp. 26–32.

8. C. Peterson and L. Bossio. "Healthy Attitudes: Optimism, Hope, and Control," in Goleman and Gurin (eds.), *Mind/Body Medicine*.

9. R. R. Wilson. *Don't Panic: Taking Control of Anxiety Attacks*. New York: Harper Perennial, 1987.

10. Norman Cousins. *Head First: The Biology of Hope*. New York: Dutton, 1989, pp. 1–3.

11. B. Moyers. *Healing and the Mind*. New York: Doubleday, 1993, pp. 195–211.

12. N. Cummings. "Somatization: When Physical Symptoms Have No Medical Cause," in Goleman and Gurin (eds.), *Mind/Body Medicine*, p. 16.

13. T. Grossbart. "The Skin: Matters of the Flesh," in Goleman and Gurin (eds.), *Mind/Body Medicine*, pp. 145–60.

14. J. C. Holland and S. Lewis. "Emotions and Cancer: What Do We Really Know?" in Goleman and Gurin (eds.), *Mind/Body Medicine*, p. 85.

15. Daniel Goleman. *Emotional Intelligence*. New York: Bantam, 1995.

16. W. Poole. *The Heart of Healing*. Atlanta: Turner, 1993, p. 85.

17. Janice Kiecolt-Glaser and Ronald Glaser. "Mind and Immunity," in Goleman and Gurin (eds.), *Mind/Body Medicine*, p. 52.

18. T. Theorell and R. H. Rahe. "Behavior and life satisfaction characteristics of Swedish subjects with myocardial infarction," *Journal of Chronic Diseases* 25 (1972), pp. 139–47.

19. Stephen S. Hall. "A Molecular Code links emotions, mind, and health," *Smithsonian* 20 (June 1989), pp. 62–71.

20. D. Goleman and J. Gurin. "What Is Mind/Body Medicine?" in Goleman and Gurin (eds.), *Mind/Body Medicine*, pp. 6–7.

21. C. Pert. "The Chemical Communicators," in Moyers, *Healing and the Mind*, p. 182.

22. J. Kiecolt-Glaser and R. Glaser. "Mind and Immunity," in Goleman and Gurin (eds.), *Mind/Body Medicine*, p. 44.

23. M. Biondi. *Acta Neurologica* 13, 4 (August 1991), p. 332.

24. R. Ornstein and D. Sobel. *Healthy Pleasures.* Reading, Mass.: Addison-Wesley, 1989, p. 27.

25. B. Justice. *Who Gets Sick?* Los Angeles: Jeremy P. Tarcher, 1987, pp. 157–58.

26. R. W. Bartrop, E. Luckhurst, L. Lazarus, L. G. Kiloh, and R. Penny. "Depressed Lymphocyte Function After Bereavement," *Lancet* 1 (8016), pp. 834–36.

27. S. E. Locke. "Stress, Adaptation, and Immunity," *General Hospital Psychiatry* 4, pp. 49–58.

28. M. Frankenhauser. "Psychobiological Aspects of Life Stress," in S. Levine and U. Holger (eds.), *Coping and Health.* New York: Plenum, pp. 203–23.

Chapter 3: Dancing with Dinosaurs and Dragons

1. These themes run through many of Miller's works, including the following: *The Drama of the Gifted Child* (New York: Basic Books, 1992); *Thou Shalt Not Be Aware: Society's Betrayal of the Child* (New York: NAL/Dutton, 1988); *The Untouched Key: Tracing Childhood Trauma in Creativity and Destructiveness* (New York: Doubleday, 1991); *Banished Knowledge: Facing Childhood Injury* (New York: Doubleday, 1991).

Chapter 4: How About a Prison Break?

1. Conversations with Joanne Murray, director of Wellesley College Center for Work and Service, January 1995.

2. Martin Seligman. *Learned Optimism.* New York: Alfred A. Knopf, 1991.

3. Ibid., pp. 218–20.

4. Ibid., pp. 178–79.

5. Susan Jeffers. *Feel the Fear and Do It Anyway.* New York: Fawcett Columbine, 1988, pp. 74–75.

6. John P. Kotter. *The New Rules: How to Succeed in Today's Post-Corporate World.* New York: Simon and Schuster, 1995, p. 199.

7. See citations for Stanley Mann, Richard Bandler, John Grinder, and Leslie Cameron-Bandler in the bibliography.

Chapter 5: *Revitalizing Your Career*

1. R. Waterman. *What America Does Right: Learning from Companies That Put People First.* New York: W. W. Norton, 1994.
2. Robert A. Ferchat. "The Chaos Factor," *The Corporate Board.* May–June 1990, p. 11.
3. "Working Flexibly," *Training and Development,* January, 1994.

Chapter 6: *Does Your Work Still Fit?*

1. C. Adelman. *Women at Thirty-Something: Paradoxes of Attainment.* Washington, D.C.: U.S. Department of Education, 1990.
2. Susan Faludi. *Backlash: The Undeclared War Against Women.* New York: Crown, 1991.
3. H. Dienstfrey. *Where the Body Meets the Mind.* New York: HarperCollins, 1992, pp. 76–77.
4. P. Howard. *The Owner's Manual for the Brain: Everyday Applications from Mind-Body Research.* Austin, Texas: Leonarian, 1994.
5. Robert Waterman, Jeffrey Pfeffer, and Tom Peters have all written extensively on the ability of organizations to increase productivity by paying close attention to the needs of their workers.
6. J. Douillard. *Body, Mind, and Sport: The Mind-Body Guide to Lifelong Fitness and Your Personal Best.* New York: Harmony, 1994, pp. 78–82.

Chapter 7: *Getting a Whole Life—Finally!*

1. *Psychology Today*, March 1994, p. 22.
2. Betty Friedan. *The Fountain of Age.* New York: Simon and Schuster, 1993.
3. C. Adelman. *Women at Thirty-Something: Paradoxes of Attainment.* Washington, D.C.: U.S. Department of Education, 1990.
4. Lydia Bronte. *The Longevity Factor: The New Reality of Long Careers and How It Can Lead to Richer Lives.* New York: HarperCollins, 1993.
5. Aaron Antonovsky. *Unraveling the Mystery of Health: How People Manage Stress and Stay Well.* San Francisco: Jossey-Bass, 1987, p. xiii.
6. Henry Dreher. *The Immune Power Personality: 7 Traits You Can Develop to Stay Healthy.* New York: Dutton, 1995, pp. 255–70.
7. H. Friedman. *Lancet* 343, January 2, 1994.

8. Larry Dossey. *Meaning and Medicine: Lessons from a Doctor's Tales of Breakthrough and Healing.* New York: Bantam Books, 1991, p. 70. Also, R. Ornstein and D. Sobel, *Healthy Pleasures.* Reading, Mass.: Addison-Wesley, 1989, p. 196.

9. *New York Times*, October 14, 1993.

10. Helen Bee. *Journey of Adulthood.* New York: Macmillan, 1987, p. 137.

11. Willis Harman and John Hormann. *Creative Work: The Constructive Role of Business in a Transforming Society.* Indianapolis: Knowledge Systems, 1990, p. 29.

12. K. Pelletier. *Sound Mind, Sound Body: A New Model for Lifelong Health.* New York: Simon and Schuster, 1994, p. 17.

13. J. Hirsch. "The Knead Is Great," *Saturday Evening Post*, January/February 1990, p. 14.

14. J. Schor. *The Overworked American: The Unexpected Decline of Leisure.* New York: Basic Books, 1992.

15. J. M. T. Finney. "Discussion of Papers on Shock," *Annals of Surgery* 100, p. 746.

16. W. N. Christenson and L. E. Hinkle. "Differences in Illness and Prognostic Signs in Two Groups of Young Men," *Journal of the American Medical Association* 177 (4), 1961, pp. 247–53.

17. J. Kiecolt-Glaser and R. Glaser. "Mind and Immunity," in Goleman and Gurin (eds.), *Mind/Body Medicine.*

18. N. Tichy. *Control Your Destiny or Someone Else Will: How Jack Welch Is Making General Electric the World's Most Competitive Company.* New York: Currency/Doubleday, 1993.

19. Godfrey, J. *Our Wildest Dreams: Women Entrepreneurs Making Money, Having Fun, Doing Good.* New York: Harper Business, 1992.

BIBLIOGRAPHY

Ader, R., Felten, D. L., and Cohen, N., eds. *Psychoneuroimmunology*, 2nd edition. San Diego: Academic Press, Harcourt Brace Jovanovich, 1991.

Adizes, Ichak. *Mastering Change: The Power of Mutual Trust and Respect in Personal Life, Family Life, Business and Society.* Santa Monica, Calif.: Adizes Institute Publications, 1991.

Antonovsky, Aaron. *Unraveling the Mystery of Health: How People Manage Stress and Stay Well.* San Francisco: Jossey-Bass, 1987.

Bailyn, Lotte. *Breaking the Mold: Women, Men and Time in the New Corporation.* New York: Free Press, 1993.

Bandler, Richard. *Using Your Brain—For a Change. Neurolinguistic Programming.* Moab, Utah: Real People, 1985.

Bandler, Richard, and Grinder, John. *Frogs Into Princes. Neurolinguistic Programming.* Moab, Utah: Real People, 1979.

———. *Reframing—Neurolinguistic Programming and the Transformation of Meaning.* Moab, Utah: Real People, 1982.

Barasch, Marc. *The Healing Path: A Soul Approach to Illness.* New York: Jeremy P. Tarcher/Putnam, 1993.

Bardwick, Judith. *Danger in the Comfort Zone: From Boardroom to Mailroom—How to Break the Entitlement Habit That's Killing American Business.* New York: Amacom, 1991.

Barrentine, Pat, ed. *When the Canary Stops Singing: Women's Perspectives on Transforming Business.* San Francisco: Berrett-Koehler, 1993.

Barnett, R., and Rivers, C. *Ozzie and Harriet Are Dead.* New York: HarperCollins, 1996.

Bepko, Claudia, and Drestan, Jo-Ann. *Singing at the Top of Our Lungs: Women, Love, and Creativity.* HarperCollins, 1993.

Blumstein, Philip, and Schwartz, Pepper. *The American Couple: Money, Work, and Sex.* New York: Morrow, 1983.

Boldt, Laurence G. *Zen and the Art of Making a Living.* New York: Arkana, 1993.

Borysenko, Joan and Miroslav. *The Power of the Mind to Heal: Renewing Body, Mind, and Spirit.* Carson, Calif.: Hay House, 1994.

Bronte, Lydia. *The Longevity Factor: The New Reality of Long Careers and How It Can Lead to Richer Lives.* New York: HarperCollins, 1993.

Burns, David, M.D. *The Feeling Good Handbook.* New York: Plume, 1989.

Buzan, Tony. *Use Both Sides of Your Brain.* New York: E. P. Dutton, 1976.

Cameron, Julia. *The Artist's Way: A Spiritual Path to Higher Creativity.* New York: Jeremy P. Tarcher, 1992.

Cameron-Bandler, Leslie, Gordon, David, and LeBeau, Michael. *Know-How: Guided Programs for Inventing Your Own Best Future.* San Rafael, Calif.: FuturePace, 1985.

Carlsen, Mary Baird. *Creative Aging: A Meaning-Making Perspective.* New York: W. W. Norton, 1991.

———. *Meaning-Making: Therapeutic Processes in Adult Development.* New York: W. W. Norton, 1988.

Chopra, Deepak. *Ageless Body, Timeless Mind: The Quantum Alternative to Growing Old.* New York: Harmony Books, 1993.

Cousins, Norman. *Head First: The Biology of Hope.* New York: E. P. Dutton, 1989.

Covey, Stephen R. *The 7 Habits of Highly Effective People: Powerful Lessons in Personal Change.* New York: Simon and Schuster, 1990.

Crosby, Faye J. *Juggling: The Unexpected Advantages of Balancing Career and Home for Women and Their Families.* New York: Free Press, 1991.

DeBono, Edward. *Serious Creativity: Using the Power of Lateral Thinking to Create New Ideas.* New York: Harper Business, 1992.

Denniston, Denise. *The TM Book: How to Enjoy the Rest of Your Life.* Fairfield, Iowa: Fairfield, 1986.

Dent, Harry S., Jr. *Job Shock: Four New Principles Transforming Our Work and Business.* New York: St. Martin's, 1995.

Dienstfrey, Harris. *Where the Body Meets the Mind.* New York: HarperCollins, 1993.

Dominguez, Joe, and Robin, Vickie. *Your Money or Your Life: Transforming Your Relationship with Money and Achieving Financial Independence.* New York: Viking Penguin, 1992.

Dossey, Larry. *Meaning and Medicine: Lessons from a Doctor's Tales of Breakthrough and Healing.* New York: Bantam, 1991.

Dotto, Lydia. *Losing Sleep: How Your Sleeping Habits Affect Your Life.* New York: William Morrow, 1990.

Douillard, John. *Body, Mind, and Sport: The Mind-Body Guide to Lifelong Fitness and Your Personal Best.* New York: Harmony, 1994.

Dreher, Henry. *The Immune Power Personality: 7 Traits You Can Develop to Stay Healthy.* New York: Dutton, 1995.

Estes, Clarissa Pinkola. *Women Who Run with the Wolves: Myths and Stories of the Wild Woman Archetype.* New York: Ballantine, 1992.

Evans, Williams, Ph.D., and Rosenberg, Irwin, M.D. *Biomarkers: The 10 Keys to Prolonging Vitality.* New York: Simon and Schuster, 1992.

Faelten, Sharon, and Diamond, David. *Take Control of Your Life: A Complete Guide to Stress Relief.* Emmaus, Pa.: Rodale, 1988.

Faludi, Susan. *Backlash: The Undeclared War Against American Women.* New York: Crown, 1991.

Fassel, Diane. *Working Ourselves to Death: The High Cost of Workaholism and the Rewards of Recovery.* San Francisco: HarperSanFrancisco, 1990.

Ferguson, Marilyn. *The Aquarian Conspiracy: Personal and Social Transformation.* Los Angeles: Jeremy P. Tarcher, 1980.

Fields, Rick. *Chop Wood Carry Water: A Guide to Finding Spiritual Fulfillment in Everyday Life.* Los Angeles: Jeremy P. Tarcher, 1984.

Flach, Frederick, M.D. *Resilience: Discovering a New Strength at Times of Stress.* New York: Fawcett Columbine, 1988.

Fletcher, Jerry L. *Patterns of High Performance: Discovering the Ways People Work Best.* San Francisco: Berrett-Koehler Publishers, 1993.

Fox, Matthew. *The Reinvention of Work: A New Vision of Livelihood for Our Time.* San Francisco: HarperCollins, 1994.

Friedan, Betty. *The Fountain of Age.* New York: Simon and Schuster, 1993.

Fritz, Robert. *The Path of Least Resistance: Learning to Become the Creative Force in Your Own Life.* New York: Fawcett Columbine, 1984.

————. *Creating.* New York: Fawcett Columbine, 1991.

Gardner, David C., and Beatty, Grace Joely. *Stop Stress and Aging Now.* Windham, N.H.: American Training and Research Association, 1985.

Gardner, Howard. *Frames of Mind: The Theory of Multiple Intelligences.* New York: Basic Books, 1993.

Gerzon, Mark. *Coming into Our Own: Understanding the Adult Metamorphosis.* New York: Delacorte, 1992.

Godfrey, Joline. *Our Wildest Dreams: Women Entrepreneurs Making Money, Having Fun, Doing Good.* New York: HarperBusiness, 1992.

Goleman, Daniel, Ph.D. *Emotional Intelligence.* New York: Bantam, 1995.

Goleman, Daniel, Ph.D., and Gurin, Joel, editors. *Mind Body Medicine: How to Use Your Mind for Better Health.* New York: Consumer Reports Books, 1993.

Goman, Carol Kinsey. *Creativity in Business: A Practical Guide for Creative Thinking.* Los Altos, Calif.: Crisp Publications, 1989.

Graham, Lawrence Otis. *The Best Companies for Minorities.* New York: Plume, 1993.

Hakim, Cliff. *We Are All Self-Employed: The New Social Contract for Working in a Changed World.* San Francisco: Berrett-Koehler, 1994.

Harman, Willis, and Hormann, John. *Creative Work: The Constructive Role of Business in a Transforming Society.* Indianapolis: Knowledge Systems, 1990.

Handy, Charles. *The Age of Unreason.* Cambridge: Harvard Business School Press, 1989.

Hanh, Thich Nhat. *Peace Is Every Step: The Path of Mindfulness in Everyday Life.* New York: Bantam, 1992.

Hawley, Jack. *Reawakening the Spirit in Work: The Power of Dharmic Management.* San Francisco: Berrett-Koehler, 1993.

Hewlett, Sylvia Ann. *When the Bough Breaks: The Cost of Neglecting Our Children.* New York: Harper Perennial, 1991.

Jeffers, Susan. *Feel the Fear and Do It Anyway.* New York: Fawcett Columbine, 1988.

Justice, Blair, Ph.D. *Who Gets Sick: How Beliefs, Moods, and Thoughts Affect Your Health.* Los Angeles: Jeremy P. Tarcher, 1987.

Kabat-Zinn, Jon. *Full Catastrophe Living: Using the Wisdom of Your Body and Mind to Face Stress, Pain, and Illness.* New York: Delacorte, 1990.

———. *Wherever You Go, There You Are.* New York: Hyperion, 1995.

Kanter, Rosabeth. *When Giants Learn to Dance: Mastering the Challenge of Strategy, Management, and Careers in the 1990s.* New York: Simon and Schuster, 1990.

Karasek, Robert. *Healthy Work: Stress, Productivity, and the Restructuring of Working Life.* New York: Basic Books, 1992.

Kaye, Yvonne, Ph.D. *Credit, Cash and Co-Dependency: The Money Connection.* Deerfield Beach, Fla.: Health Communications, 1991.

Kotter, John P. *The New Rules: How to Succeed in Today's Post-Corporate World.* New York: Simon and Schuster, 1995.

Krannich, Ronald L., Ph.D. *Change Your Job/Change Your Life: High Impact Strategies for Finding Great Jobs in the 90's.* Manassas Park, Va.: Impact Publications, 1994.

LaBier, Douglas. *Modern Madness. The Emotional Fall-out of Success.* Reading, Mass.: Addison-Wesley, 1986.

Langer, Ellen, Ph.D. *Mindfulness.* Lawrence, Mass.: Addison-Wesley, 1989.

Levering, Robert. *A Great Place to Work.* New York: Random House, 1988.

Levine, Barbara Hoberman. *Your Body Believes Every Word You Say: The Language of the Body/Mind Connection.* Lower Lake, Calif.: Aslan, 1991.

Lynch, James P., D.C. *Dr. Lynch's Holistic Self-Health Program: Three Months to Total Well-Being.* New York: Dutton, 1994.

Maddi, Salvatore R., and Kobasa, Suzanne C. *The Hardy Executive: Health Under Stress.* Chicago: Dow-Jones-Irwin, 1984.

Mann, Stanley. *Triggers: A New Approach to Self-Motivation.* Englewood Cliffs, N.J.: Prentice-Hall, 1987.

McAdams, Dan. *Power, Intimacy, and the Life Story.* Chicago: Dorsey, 1985.

McGee-Cooper, Ann, Trammell, Duane, and Lau, Barbara. *You Don't Have to Go Home from Work Exhausted.* New York: Bantam, 1990.

Melohn, Tom. *The New Partnership: Profit by Bringing Out the Best in Your People.* Essex Junction, Vt.: Oliver Wight, 1994.

Miller, Alice. *The Drama of the Gifted Child.* New York: Basic Books, 1983.

———. *Thou Shalt Not Be Aware: Society's Betrayal of the Child.* New York: NAL/Dutton, 1988.

———. *The Untouched Key: Tracing Childhood Trauma in Creativity and Destructiveness.* New York: Anchor, 1990.

———. *Breaking Down the Wall of Silence: The Liberating Experience of Facing the Painful Truth.* New York: NAL/Dutton, 1993.

Moore, Thomas, Ph.D. *Care of the Soul: A Guide for Cultivating Depth and Sacredness in Everyday Life.* New York: Harper Perennial, 1992.

Moyers, Bill. *Healing and the Mind.* New York: Doubleday, 1993.

Noer, David M. *Healing the Wounds: Overcoming the Trauma of Layoffs and Revitalizing Downsized Organizations.* San Francisco: Jossey-Bass, 1993.

Northrup, Christanne, M.D. *Women's Bodies, Women's Wisdom.* New York: Bantam, 1994.

Ornish, Dean, M.D. *Program for Reversing Heart Disease.* New York: Random House, 1990.

Ornstein, Robert, and Sobel, David. *Healthy Pleasures.* Reading, Mass.: Addison-Wesley, 1989.

Osherson, Samuel. *Finding Our Fathers: The Unfinished Business of Manhood.* New York: Free Press, 1986.

Peck, M. Scott, M.D. *A World Waiting to Be Born: Civility Rediscovered.* New York: Bantam, 1993.

Pelletier, Kenneth R. *Sound Mind, Sound Body: A New Model for Lifelong Health.* New York: Simon and Schuster, 1994.

Peters, Tom. *Liberation Management. Necessary Disorganization for the Nanosecond Nineties.* New York: Alfred A. Knopf, 1992.

Pfeffer, Jeffrey. *Competitive Advantage Through People: Unleashing the Power of the Work Force.* Cambridge, Mass.: Harvard Business School Press, 1994.

Pierce, J. Howard. *The Owner's Manual for the Brain: Everyday Applications from Mind-Brain Research.* Austin, Tex.: Leonarian, 1994.

Poole, William, and the Institute for Noetic Sciences. *The Heart of Healing.* Atlanta: Turner, 1993.

Ray, Michael, and Rinzler, Alan. *The New Paradigm in Business: Emerging Strategies for Leadership and Organizational Change.* Los Angeles: Jeremy P. Tarcher, 1993.

Robinson, Bryan. *Overdoing It: How to Slow Down and Take Care of Yourself.* Health Communications, 1992.

Rosen, Robert. *The Healthy Company: Eight Strategies to Develop People, Productivity, and Products.* Los Angeles: Jeremy P. Tarcher, 1991.

Saltzman, Amy. *Downshifting. Reinventing Success on a Slower Track.* New York: HarperCollins, 1991.

Schor, Juliet. *The Overworked American: The Unexpected Decline of Leisure.* New York: Basic Books, 1992.

Schwartz, Felice N. (with Jean Zimmerman). *Breaking with Tradition: Women and Work, The New Facts of Life.* New York: Time Warner, 1992.

Seligman, Martin. *Learned Optimism.* New York: Alfred A. Knopf, 1991.

Senge, Peter. *The Fifth Discipline: The Art and Practice of the Learning Organization.* New York: Doubleday, 1990.

Shealy, C. Norman, and Myss, Carolyn. *The Creation of Health: The Emotional, Psychological, and Spiritual Responses that Promote Health and Healing*. Walpole, N.H.: Stillpoint, 1993.

Sheehy, Gail. *New Passages: Mapping Your Life Across Time*. New York: Random House, 1995.

Sher, Barbara. *I Could Do Anything If I Only Knew What It Was: How To Discover What You Really Want and How to Get It*. New York: Delacorte, 1994.

Sinetar, Marsha. *To Build the Life You Want, Create the Work You Love: The Spiritual Dimension of Entrepreneuring*. New York: St. Martin's, 1995.

Stack, Jack. *The Great Game of Business: The Only Sensible Way to Run a Company*. New York: Doubleday, 1992.

Steinem, Gloria. *Revolution from Within: A Book of Self-Esteem*. Boston: Little, Brown, 1992.

Tichy, Noel M., and Sherman, Stratford. *Control Your Destiny or Someone Else Will: How Jack Welch Is Making General Electric the World's Most Competitive Company*. New York: Doubleday, 1993.

Waterman, Robert H. *What America Does Right: Learning from Companies That Put People First*. New York: W. W. Norton, 1994.

Weil, Andrew, M.D. *Health and Healing*. Boston: Houghton Mifflin, 1983.

———. *Spontaneous Healing: How to Discover and Enhance Your Body's Natural Ability to Maintain and Heal Itself*. New York: Alfred A. Knopf, 1995.

Weisbord, Marvin. *Productive Workplaces: Organizing and Managing for Dignity, Meaning, and Community*. San Francisco: Jossey-Bass, 1991.

Wheatley, Margaret. *Leadership and the New Science: Learning About Organization from an Orderly Universe*. San Francisco: Berrett-Koehler, 1993.

Whitmyer, Claude. *Mindfulness and Meaningful Work: Explorations in Right Livelihood*. Berkeley, Calif.: Parallax, 1994.

Whyte, David. *The Heart Aroused: Poetry and the Preservation of the Soul in Corporate America*. New York: Doubleday, 1994.

Wilson, R. Reid, Ph.D. *Don't Panic: Taking Control of Anxiety Attacks*. New York: Harper Perennial, 1987.

Wonder, Jacquelyn, and Donovan, Priscilla. *The Flexibility Factor: Why People Who Thrive on Change Are Successful and How You Can Become One of Them*. New York: Doubleday, 1989.

Woronoff, John. *The Japanese Management Mystique: The Reality Behind the Myth*. Burr Ridge, Ill.: Irwin Professional Publishing, 1994.

Wujec, Tom. *Pumping Ions: Games and Exercises to Flex Your Mind.* New York: Doubleday, 1988.

Wycoff, Joyce. *Mindmapping: Your Personal Guide to Exploring Creativity and Problem-Solving.* New York: Berkley, 1991.

INDEX

· A NOTE ON THE TYPE ·

The typeface used in this book is a version of Times Roman, originally designed by Stanley Morison (1889–1967), the scholar who supervised Monotype's revivals of classic typefaces (Bembo) and commisioned new ones from Eric Gill (Perpetua), among others. Having censured *The Times* of London in an article, Morison was challenged to better it. Taking Plantin as a basis, he sought to produce a typeface that would be classical but not dull, compact without looking cramped, and would keep high readability on a range of papers. "*The Times* New Roman" debuted on October 3, 1932, and was almost instantly in great demand; it has become perhaps the most widely used of all typefaces (though the paper changed typeface again in 1972). Given its success, it is noteworthy that it was Morison's only original design. Ironically, he had pangs of conscience, writing later, "[William] Morris would have denounced [it]."